Solving the Interstitial Cystitis Puzzle

My Story of Discovery and Recovery

Amrit K. Willis, RN, BSN

Holistic Life Enterprises

Los Angeles

Published by

Holistic Life Enterprises
9461 Charleville Boulevard
Suite 198
Beverly Hills, CA 90212

Design and Layout by
MICROGLYPHICS

Library of Congress Catalogue Number: 2001090105

International Standard Book Numbers (ISBN):

Cloth: 0-9710869-0-7

Paper: 0-9710869-1-5

Electronic (PDF): 0-9710869-4-X

Printed in the United States of America

Dedication

This book is dedicated to all those individuals who suffer from interstitial cystitis. May you find hope and inspiration in your healing.

May all beings be happy.

May all beings be free from suffering.

Acknowledgements

I wish to thank God and my parents for giving me life.

I would like to thank Julian Lange and Dr. Roger Barnes in helping in my discovery and recovery from interstitial cystitis.

I wish to express my deepest love to my precious son, Hunter.

I want to give my most profound gratitiude and love to my dearest husband, without whose help this book could not have been completed. His love, patience, and devotion to my welfare is deeply appreciated. I am truly blessed.

Last but not least, I wish to express my deepest gratitude to Dr. Allen Weiner, for without his loving patience and guidance this book would have never been written.

Disclaimer

PLEASE READ THE DISCLAIMER CAREFULLY BEFORE USING THIS BOOK. By using this book, you signify your assent to this disclaimer. If you do not agree to this disclaimer, please do not use the book.

Amrit K. Willis, RN, BSN, is a holistic nurse not a medical doctor. I am a recovered IC patient sharing my discovery and recovery from IC. Statements made are not intended to diagnose, treat, cure, or prevent any disease. This information is not intended to replace the advice, diagnosis, or treatment of a medical doctor. The information in this book is for educational and research purposes, and neither the author nor publisher intends to provide medical diagnosis or medical treatment.

Any attempt to diagnose and treat an illness using the information in this book should come under the direction of a holistic medical physician. Because there is always some risk involved in any treatment or procedure, the publisher and author are not responsible for any adverse effects or consequences resulting from the use of any of the suggestions or procedures in this book.

Anyone seeking to take any of the supplements and therapies mentioned in this book should do so only under the care and advice of a holistic medical doctor, holistic naturopath, or other competent, licensed health care professional. Please do not use this book if you are unwilling to assume the risks. In the event you use this information without your doctor's approval, you are prescribing for yourself, which is your constitutional right.

You can find a holistic medical doctor by going to http://www.acam.org/doctorsearch.php for the American College for Advancement in Medicine or call (800) 532-3688.

CONTENTS

Solving the Interstitial Cystitis Puzzle

Contents 13

PREFACE

"Until man can produce a blade of grass, nature can laugh at his so called scientific knowledge. Remedies from chemicals will never stand in favour compared with the products of nature, the living cell of the plant and the final result of the rays of the sun, the mother of all life."

— Thomas A. Edison

The purpose of this book is to share with those individuals who are suffering from interstitial cystitis (IC) my discoveries and recovery from this painful *dis*-ease. Briefly, through my research, studies, and my own healing process with IC, it became apparent that I had an acid-alkali imbalance—, that a person with IC is in an acidic state.

"I believe that our differences arise out of our one major commonality, which in my opinion is this...

"IC patients have a toxic body.

"We are all toxic for different reasons and to different degrees, but I have found that IC patients have pretty much the epitome of the toxic body. The more severe the IC the more toxic and sick the rest of the body. IC patients often feel as if they are full of poison or on chemical overload. There is a feeling of too much acid in the system. (This is why antacids, baking soda and water, Prelief™, and Tummy Tamers are so helpful to many IC patients. They allow them to be able to eat and drink things they normally couldn't tolerate, providing them some relief from the pain and burning.) The stomach, the intestines, the kidneys and bladder are all burning with acid. This is what

IC felt like to me and to many other IC patients I have spoken to." [1]

Reports from the medical community show that individuals with IC complain that acidic foods and beverages cause an exacerbation of symptoms, such as pain and burning in the bladder. It has also been reported by the medical community that taking alkalizing substances, such as baking soda as a supplement or Prelief™ sprinkled on food, diminishes IC symptoms. What this indicates to me is that persons with IC need to decrease the body's acidity and increase alkalinity.

Most Americans are eating an inverted diet of 80% **acid-forming** foods and only 20% **alkali-forming** foods.

In Dr. Susan Lark's book *The Chemistry of Success*, she examined the Economic Research Service of the USDA statistics of the American diet. She added up the number of pounds of highly acid-forming foods that the average American eats per year with the average yearly intake of more alkali-forming foods. The ratio she discovered was 17:3 in favor of acid-forming foods. This highly acid-forming diet puts a great strain on the buffering systems of the body to neutralize all the acid that is produced by such a diet.

Dr. Lark states, "As we age, our ability to maintain a slightly alkaline balance in our cells and tissues diminishes. All too many factors in modern life, including the standard American diet, also affect acid-alkali balance in the body. Our diet is high in acidic and acid-creating foods, and the fast pace of life today increases acidity." [2]

"Maintaining the cells and tissues of the body in their healthy, slightly alkaline state helps to prevent inflammation. In contrast, over acidity promotes the onset of painful and disabling inflammatory conditions as diverse as colds, sinusitis, rheumatoid arthritis and interstitial cystitis." [3]

"The body does not have an endless quantity of bicarbonate ions available to neutralize all irresponsible infringements on the law of alkaline-acid. The alkaline reserve is only a back-up system with limited quantity to keep you from constantly poisoning yourself with too much acid-forming food. When there is overindulgence in acid-forming foods (especially fried processed foods), the body sickens. In its marvelous wisdom, the body will make every possible effort to rebalance this transgression by expelling as quickly as possible, all the acid-forming residues. But when this alkaline reserve is depleted, death follows." [4]

In this book, I will define interstitial cystitis and present demographics and the history of some acid-alkali studies. I will also review the anatomy of the bladder and briefly discuss some current treatments for IC. I will explain acid-alkali balance and how to measure your body's pH. I will discuss the leaky gut syndrome (LGS) and its relationship to allergies and inflammatory conditions. I will also present the following topics relative to IC: liver flush, osteoporosis, hormones, sex, alkali-forming diet, alkaline water, meal suggestions, lifestyle alternatives, and supplements.

It was only a matter of few days before I started to feel better on the alkali-forming diet. Just like a diabetic checks their blood sugar levels and alters their diet I was able to monitor my own progress by measuring the pH of my urine and correcting my diet.

By changing to an alkali-forming diet/lifestyle, eliminating foods and environmental factors to which I was allergic, and addressing the leaky gut syndrome, I was able to gain control over my own healing process.

"Modern medicine teaches that pain means sickness. It does not recognize that pain is also the body's way of informing us that we are doing something wrong. Pain can tell us that we are smoking too much, eating too much, or eating the wrong things." [5]

[1] Catherine M. Simone, *Along the Healing Path, Recovering from Interstitial Cystitis*, Kearney, NE: Morris Publishing, 2000, pp. 6 - 7

[2] Dr. Susan Lark, MD, and James A. Richards, MBA, *The Chemistry of Success*, San Francisco: Bay Books, 2000, p. 55

[3] *Ibid.*

[4] Dr. Theodore A. Baroody, Jr., MA, DC, ND, PhD, *Alkalize or Die*, Waynesville, NC: Eclectic Press, 1993, pp. 21-22

[5] Linda G. Rector-Page, ND, PhD, *Healthy Healing, 9th*, Carmel Valley: Healthy Healing Publications, 1992, p. 9

TESTIMONIAL

"There are three categories of drugs; the lowest one of which is poison, the second one is a little poisonous, the highest one is no poison. The lowest drug cures six out of ten sicknesses, leaving poisons in the patient. The middle one cures seven out of ten sicknesses, leaving a small amount of poison. Even the highest medicine can only cure eight or nine out of ten sicknesses. The sicknesses that medicine cannot cure can be cured only by foods."

— The Nei Ching

My journey of interstitial cystitis began in 1996. I experienced multiple bouts of cystitis that summer and fall, and took several courses of broad-spectrum antibiotics. In January of 1997 at the age of 44, I became pregnant.

Not long after my son's birth, I began to experience more episodes of pain and urinary frequency, usually resorting to taking more antibiotics. I sought the help of acupuncturists, herbalists, chiropractors, yoga, gynecologists, and urologists.

As is typical of most IC patients, I endured several years of suffering and seeking numerous medical consults until I was finally diagnosed with IC. I was worn out and depressed from the burning and pain in my bladder, nocturia (night time urinary frequency), and urinating every 5 to 10 minutes during the day.

Consulting yet another urologist's office, my urine specimen was sterile. There was no infection. He performed a cystoscopy and informed me I had interstitial cystitis. I was very upset. I was told by the urologist I could come into the doctor's office and have medications or steroids injected into my bladder on a regular basis. He said the cause and cure of IC was unknown but certain oral medications might help relieve some pain.

Then my urologist gave me my first glimmer of hope. He handed me a simple diet sheet with a few foods to avoid and said that by eliminating these certain foods I might decrease some of my pain. It was apparent to me that if avoiding certain foods helped diminish the symptoms of IC that the answer to its resolution was diet-related.

Returning home, I explored my holistic books and references, and I searched for an answer to my healing. I found the suggestions I had tried before, such as; uva-ursi, tinctures of corn silk, marshmallow leaf, golden seal, cranberry juice, acupressure points, relaxation techniques, sitz baths, heating pads, cold packs et cetera. These were supportive but not a cure. I turned to *Alternative Medicine: The Definitive Guide* by the Burton Goldberg Group. Something Dr. Larrian Gillespie , MD, stated about diet and cystitis struck me, "If you have an infection, taking cranberry juice, which contains hippuronic acid, makes as much sense as putting out a fire with gasoline, it only adds more acid to the urine, which in turn, increases the burning sensation. Cranberry juice may be helpful if you want to prevent an infection, but if you already have one, it only makes matters worse. Rather, try one-quarter teaspoon of baking soda in water. You should feel relief in twenty minutes." [1]

My urologist was suggesting diet modifications. Dr. Gillespie was suggesting a dose of baking soda that I knew would increase one's pH. These were things I could research and control. To me, this added up to examining my diet and assessing my pH or acid-alkali balance. I was intrigued. I checked my urine pH; it was 4.6. Normal urine has a pH of 4.6 to 8. Wine has a pH of 3.5. Could it be my urine was burning my bladder? I recall over the years feeling as if I was "allergic" to my own urine. Urinating or getting rid of the urine gave some temporary relief.

I needed to raise the pH of my urine—, but how? I needed to explore also the possibility of allergies to food and my environment. My next stop was Santa Monica Homeopathic Pharmacy where I discovered a book entitled *Acid and Alkaline* by Herman Aihara. Here are some following excerpts that convinced me to experiment with an alkali-forming diet: "Most proteins in food combine with sulfur and many are also combined with phosphorus. When the protein is metabolized, these elements remain as sulfuric acid and phosphoric acid and must be neutralized by ammonia, calcium, sodium, and potassium before they can be excreted by the kidneys. This is the reason high protein foods, especially animal foods, generally are acid forming foods. This is also true of most grains because they contain much sulfur and phosphorus. In fruit and most vegetables, the organic acid (such as the acidity of an orange which you can taste) contains many elements such as potassium, sodium, calcium, and magnesium. Organic acids, when oxidized, become carbon dioxide and water; the alkaline elements (K, Na, Ca, Mg) remain and neutralize body acid. In other words, strangely enough, acid foods reduce body acids. This is the reason that fruits and most vegetables are considered alkaline forming foods. Conversely, high protein foods and most grains, when metabolized, produce acid that must be neutralized; therefore they are generally acid forming foods." [2]

"In theory, whether a given food is acid forming or alkaline forming is determined by the proportion of acid forming and alkaline forming elements contained in the food. In practical reality, however, it is determined by test tube. This procedure is known as titration. First, the food to be measured is burned to ashes. (It is this step of burning the food that takes the place of digestion and thus gives us a picture of whether the food is acid or alkaline forming.) Next, a standard amount of very pure water, say one liter, is added to 100 grams of these ashes to make a solution. This solution is tested to see whether it is acid or alkaline. Once we know whether the solution is acid or alkaline, we can measure the concentration or strength of the acidity or alkalinity of the ash solution." [3]

After assessing my diet, I realized I was eating a high protein, acid-forming diet and probably consuming foods known to cause allergies for me. I never considered I might have had food allergies, but as I recalled there were times over the years the inner corners of my eyes became irritated and red after eating, and I had bouts of sneezing. The irritation went away after some time. I assumed I was allergic to pollen or a blooming plant.

I eliminated coffee, spices and other bladder irritants from my diet and made an appointment to be checked for food allergies with my holistic health care provider. We started a list of foods I was allergic to: potatoes, wheat, peanuts, and rice. These were some of my favorite foods and the ones I preferred to eat.

I started a list of alkali-forming foods I was not allergic to and consumed only those foods. For the next several days, I ate only foods listed on the alkali-forming allergy-free diet list: broccoli, carrots, spinach, tofu, apple juice, vanilla yogurt, and almonds. In the first forty-eight hours of converting to an alkali-forming diet, I did note some periods of poor concentration, but this soon passed. You may find your mental capacities to react or respond slower in the first 24 to 48 hours of switching to an alkali-forming diet, but this will clear. You may even want to consider starting an alkaline program on the weekend because of this possible side effect.

Within several days of starting the diet, I noted a marked decrease in my urgency and frequency to urinate. To my amazement, my pain and burning was disappearing. I checked my urine pH. 7 is a neutral pH. My urine pH had changed from 4.6 to 5.5. This might seem like an insignificant change, but the change of one point using the pH scale indicated my urine was ten times more alkaline. I was urinating every 2 hours instead of every 10 minutes. I was only getting up at night once to urinate instead of my usual every two hours.

It took months of trial and error of adding, assessing, and eliminating certain foods, beverages, and spices. I kept a food and bladder-pain and pH diary to document my findings. I lost some weight and felt more energized.

I was usually pain-free unless I encountered a food to which I was allergic. When I did run into a food that caused me pain or burning, I had to wait many hours to have it fade away until I discovered taking a homeopathic remedy for allergies and inflammation eliminated my pain in 15 to 20 minutes. Taking the homeopathic for allergies after I had a food reaction really hastened my assessment process.

During this assessment period, I did not use any perfumes and took no over the counter medications. I took no supplements, vitamins, or herbs. I used a natural organic soap and shampoo to which I was not allergic. I drank distilled water and apple juice. I drink alkaline water now—more about that later.

Since much of my diet consisted of organic vegetables, some fruits low in citric acid, apple juice, vanilla yogurt, tofu, and almonds, I was not worried about my nutrition score. I chose fresh organic foods whenever possible. I started with mostly vegetables because I found them to be less troublesome than citrus fruits.

When on an allergy elimination diet and testing for allergies, one is in a state of calorie restriction. When one is in a state of calorie restriction the urine pH will be lower, so until one can reach the daily calorie requirements for weight maintenance the urine pH may be decreased. Do not be discouraged if your urine pH is lower in the beginning. An alkalizing program can take one to two years for the body to regain its balance and build an alkali reserve again. However, you should start to feel the benefits of an alkali-forming diet combined with allergy elimination diet within a few days.

By eating an alkali-forming allergy-free diet with adequate calories, one should see the trend of the urine pH begin to rise. After several months on the alkali-forming allergy-free diet, my morning urine pH trend was 6.5 to 7.

I am still adding foods as of this writing like legumes, additional fruits, spices, et cetera. It has taken several months to determine what alkali-forming allergy-free foods to eat and what personal care items were allergy-free.

Once establishing the alkali-forming allergy-free food list, one can add new foods as time passes watching for symptoms. What I discovered was that the better alkalized I became my tolerance for foods that originally bothered me improved. For example, originally I could not tolerate juices or fruits high in citric acid, such as oranges, lemons, pineapple or spicy foods. After a few months on the alkali-forming diet, I have no problem eating citrus fruits or even spicy foods. (And I am *not* using alkalizing supplements to tolerate these foods.) Guacamole is one of my favorite alkalizing foods since it contains tomatoes and avocadoes, which are high in potassium. I added perfume, supplements, vitamins, herbs, et cetera, one at a time after I was comfortable and observed for any IC symptoms.

It is a time-consuming process, but I am determined to live pain-free without drugs or frequent medical intervention.

While searching for an answer to solving my interstitial cystitis puzzle, I found there was an underlying acid-alkali imbalance. However, since the body systems are interconnected

I discovered that I needed to address other systems that had to be restored because they were also affecting my inflammation, discomfort, and acid-alkali imbalance.

I took multiple courses of antibiotics over the years for my history of cystitis, which in turn destroyed the normal healthy flora in my gastro-intestinal tract. When the "good" bacteria are wiped out with antibiotics one can develop what is now classified in the medical community as the leaky gut syndrome (LGS.) LGS allows large food particles to leak into the blood stream, which causes the body's immune system to see these food particles as foreign, and responds by releasing histamine, which causes an inflammatory response, i.e., food allergies. Any inflammatory process will increase a person's acidity.

In addition, LGS causes malnutrition and pH imbalance because nutrients are not being absorbed properly. Large food particles in the blood stream also puts additional stress on the liver since blood carrying nutrients from the small intestines goes directly through the blood portal system to the liver. Therefore, in resolving IC I looked holistically at my recovery.

My symptoms of cystitis were treated with antibiotics. In turn, these antibiotics eventually lead to a weakening and leakage of the intestines or LGS. LGS leads to multiple food allergies and its accompanying inflammation, malnutrition, and an overtaxed liver.

The first and most important step in my recovery from IC was to switch to an alkali-forming diet, which will be discussed in the following chapters. LGS, food allergies, a liver flush, stress and nutrition needed to be addressed.

Alleluia! Now I could take my little son to a park even if it did not have a bathroom! I was ecstatic, and so was my husband. I decided to research this subject further, and knew I wanted to write a book explaining this puzzle and my discoveries and my recovery from IC.

[1] Burton Goldberg Group, *Alternative Medicine: The Definitive Guide,* Puyallup, WA: Future Medicine Publishing, 1993, p. 669

[2] Herman Aihara, *Acid and Alkaline, 5th Edition*, Oroville, CA: George Ohsawa Macrobiotic Foundation, 1986, .p. 23

[3] *Ibid.* p. 36

DEFINING INTERSTITIAL CYSTITIS

Interstitial: Relating to or situated in the small, narrow spaces between tissues or parts of an organ

Cystitis: Inflammation of the urinary bladder

"Interstitial cystitis (IC) is characterized by urgency, frequency, nocturia, and bladder pain that is generally relieved by voiding. The urine is sterile, and the urine cytology shows no evidence of malignancy. In 1915, Hunner reported on eight women with a history of suprapubic pain, frequency, nocturia, and urgency. Cystoscopically, he described either linear cracks in the bladder wall or ulcers (Hunner, 1915). At that time, he concluded 'a diagnosis of this peculiar form of bladder ulceration depends ultimately on its resistance to all ordinary forms of treatment.'

"Thus, IC was a diagnosis of exclusion in 1915 and remains so today."[1] The article continues, "The endothelial surface of the transitional cells lining the bladder has a surface mucus coat that in part contains glycosaminoglycans (GAG). The so-called GAG layer consists of mucopolysaccharides attached to a core protein that in turn is bound to a central hyaluronic acid string (Ratcliffe, 1994) Parsons et al. (1977) have shown the GAG layer to be involved in the defense mechanisms of the bladder urothelium. The glycosaminoglycans in the epithelium are distinct from those of deeper layers, implying a different function (Hurst et al., 1987). This bladder surface can be digested with *acid*, after which there is an increase in the adherence of bacteria, proteins, and calcium to the bladder epithelium. (Parsons et al., 1985, 1980)" [2]

When exploring the possibility of IC, make certain that you are examined by a gynecologist as well as a urologist. Other medical problems that have similar symptoms to IC need to be ruled out and/or treated such as: vaginitis or vaginal infections that can cause pain and burning from yeast, trichomonas, bacterial vaginosis, and herpes. Some other problems that can cause similar symptoms to IC include: bladder infections or bacterial cystitis and benign and malignant bladder tumors. In addition, endometriosis, hernias, and scar tissue from a C-section could be causing complications as well. A chiropractic evaluation is prudent since spinal misalignments can put pressure on the nerves innervating the bladder and cause pain. All these possibilities need to be considered and resolved if present.

Dr. Larrian Gillespie, MD, uro-gynecologist, and former medical director of the Pelvic Pain Treatment Center in Beverly Hills, California, has written a book titled *You Don't Have to Live with Cystitis*. She is a medical expert in this field and has treated thousands of patients with interstitial cystitis.

In describing IC, Dr. Gillespie states, "It involves…a slow destruction of the bladder by urine." [3] "Urine, with all its toxic substances and high acidity, does not burn or injure a normal bladder. But if you constantly put urine directly on skin that has no protective GAG layer, you will get a burn." [4] "Urine is indeed ulcerating and could burn away the very lining of the bladder." [5] "As I developed a model, a patient one day told me she was taking baking soda for her symptoms and found it helpful…Baking soda is alkaline. It would make the urine in the kidney less acid… In turn, urine reaching the bladder would be less acid and therefore less highly charged." [6]

Dr. Gillespie goes on to address the urine pH factor of

the IC patients she has worked with. She states her patients' urine in the **bladder** was found to be alkaline or in other words with a higher pH. She attributes a higher urine pH to the fact that cells in the bladder leak bicarbonate to compensate for the bladder tissues being burned by urine that had a low or acidic pH. She confirms that her IC patients had a low urine pH because the urine she evaluated by catheterization from the **kidneys** was 5.5. (Normal urine pH is 4.6 to 8. A pH below 7 using the pH scale is acidic, while a pH above 7 is alkaline.)

Before starting the alkali-forming diet, my urine pH was 4.6. Urine pH fluctuates throughout the day depending on diet and activity. My urine pH was consistently below 6 during my assessment process, indicating my body was excreting excess acid.

It is known that the bladder of a person with long time IC is shrunken and shriveled. Damage to the susceptible bladder might be caused by acidic urine along with bladder toxins and irritants, allergies and its related inflammation, and an overall acidic state with decreased blood and oxygen circulation to the bladder.

By maintaining a higher blood pH with an alkali-forming diet/lifestyle, one may maintain a healthy alkaline blood pH, maintain a healthy alkaline state for tissues and organs with proper circulation of nutrients and oxygen, and get a more neutral urine pH that will not injure the bladder. Generally, when the urine pH is 6.0 and below for extended periods of time it is an indication that the body fluids elsewhere are too acidic, and the body is working to rid itself of an acid medium. The bladder breaks down after years of decreased circulation related to acidic tissues and exposure to overly acidic urine.

Not every person who has an acid-forming diet has IC. However, many individuals have other inflammatory processes such as colitis, arthritis, prostatitis, cholecystitis (gall bladder disease), et cetera. What this suggests is that symptoms of inflammation and pain can manifest differently based upon an individual's weak links. In persons with IC, one of the weak links is the bladder.

Living in an acid state is not good for the human body. There appear to be several other mitigating factors that may have weakened the bladder in persons with IC. With respect to children and adolescents, the following history might predispose them to IC:

Overuse of antibiotics, usually related to multiple childhood ear infections, contributes to LGS.

LGS predisposes one to food allergies and inflammation. Food allergies and its related inflammatory state contribute to acidosis.

Childhood asthma, a compromised respiratory condition, can contribute to an acidic state.

Immature bodies and organs are sensitive and cannot tolerate highly acidic diet/lifestyle.

Each case should be evaluated individually.

Acidic urine bathes the bladder almost continuously due to the general acid-forming diet most Americans consume. In addition to an acid-forming diet, Americans also consume medications and over the counter drugs that are toxic and acidic to the bladder and add insult to injury.

My exacerbation of symptoms of burning, frequency and pain were related to the consumption of acid-forming foods, highly acidic foods, substances that were toxic and irritating to the bladder, and certain allergens that I was exposed to, usually in food. These were all irritants to a compromised and sensitive bladder.

It has been documented that the elimination of certain acidic foods and substances (like cola with a pH of 2.5) for persons with IC and the addition of an alkaline substance sodium bicarbonate (baking soda with a pH of 8.3) could help diminish the symptoms of pain and burning. What this indicates is the need to decrease acid and increase the alkali in our bodies.

[1] Meredith F. Campbell (Editor), *Campbell's Urology, Update 14,* W. B. Saunders, Co., 1995, p. 1

[2] *Ibid.* p. 5

[3] Dr. Larrian Gillespie, MD, *You Don't Have to Live with Cystitis,* New York: Avon, 1996, p. 57

[4] *Ibid.* p. 65

[5] *Ibid.* p. 67

[6] *Ibid.* p. 66

DEMOGRAPHICS

"The best prescription is knowledge."

— Dr. C. Everett Koop, former Surgeon General of the US

The demographics of this condition are as follows: from an article taken from Campbell's Urology "The majority of patients with IC are female. Koziol (1994), in a survey of 565 IC patients, reported that 89 per cent were female. The age of onset is variable, with the reported median age at onset of the IC symptoms between 40 and 50 years of age, with 9% to 26% of patients under 30 at onset of symptoms. (Held, 1994) Hanash and Pool (1970) reported a peak incidence between 60 and 69 for men in their series. The IC syndrome has been reported in children and adolescents. (Farkas et al., 1977; Geist and Antolak, 1970)." [1]

Dr. Gillespie states, "In England, for example, it has been found in 1 of every 660 outpatients with cystitis. In Scandinavia, it has been identified in 1 in 350 patients. In the United States, some physicians believe that 1 in 20 cystitis sufferers is a victim of interstitial cystitis. If interstitial cystitis is an environmental disease, such variations in incidence are to be expected. Women in Europe are exposed to different drugs, pollution factor, and diets from American women." [2]

"I don't want to belabor you with statistics, but suffice it to say that the harder we look for patients with this disease, the more we find. It is estimated now that there are probably close to 1,000,000 people whom we have already diagnosed with IC. This is just the tip of the iceberg. The more we spread the word and the more we educate our primary care doctors and gynecologists, the more patients we will be able to find and, most importantly, the more patients we will be able to help." [3]

[1] Campbell, *Op. Cit., p. 3*

[2] Gillespie, *Op. Cit.*, p. 58

[3] http://www.centralparkurology.com/services.shtml

FOUNDATION OF ACID-ALKALI IMBALANCE

"Evident facts having an unorthodox appearance are suppressed."

— Dr. Alexis Carrel

The following individuals and the research they pursued help to support my understanding of the importance of maintaining a proper acid-alkali balance in the body.

Dr. Alexia Carrel, MD

Alexia Carrel, 1912 Nobel prizewinner, surgeon, and physiologist, kept a chicken heart alive for about thirty years. He incubated a chicken egg. The heart of the developing young chick was taken out and cut in pieces. These pieces, consisting of many cells, were transferred into a saline solution that contained minerals in the same proportion as chicken blood. He changed this solution everyday, and he kept the chick's heart alive for about thirty years. When he stopped changing this solution, the heart cells died. The secret of the chick's heart surviving so many years lies in the fact that he kept the extra cellular fluids constant and that he disposed of the acidic cellular waste products every day by changing the fluid in which the chick's heart was kept. Cells will deteriorate when acid waste products accumulate.

Dr. Otto Warburg

In 1931, German biochemist, Dr. Otto Warburg, won his first Nobel Prize for work proving cancer is caused by a lack of oxygen in the cells. He states in *The Prime Cause and Prevention of Cancer* that the cause of cancer is no longer a mystery; we know it occurs whenever any cell is denied 60% of its oxygen requirements. This occurs through a buildup of pollution or toxicity within and around the cell that blocks and then damages the cellular oxygen respiration mechanism. In 1944, he won a second Nobel Prize for his work linking cancer to damaged cell respiration due to a lack of oxygen at the cellular level.

In his book, *The Metabolism of Tumors*, [1] Dr. Warburg demonstrates that the primary cause of cancer was the replacement of oxygen, an alkaline element, in the respiratory chemistry of normal cells by the fermentation of sugar, an acidic environment. The growth of cancer cells is a fermentation process that can be initiated only in the relative absence of oxygen.

Dr. Keichi Morishita, MD

"According to Keichi Morishita, MD, in his *Hidden Truth of Cancer*, [2] if the blood develops a more acidic condition, then our body inevitably deposits these excess acidic substances in some area of the body such so that the blood will be able to maintain an alkaline condition. As this tendency continues, such areas increase in acidity and some cells die; then these dead cells themselves turn into acids. However, some other cells may adapt in that environment. In other words, instead of dying, as normal cells do in an acid environment, some cells survive by becoming abnormal cells. These abnormal cells are called malignant cells. This is cancer. In other words, a deficiency of oxygen (an alkaline element) in human cells in an acid environment is the cause of cancer growth." [3]

Herman Aihara

"Why does an acidic condition in the body fluids cause cells to become malignant? Acidity in the extracellular fluids kills nerve cells which are connected with the brain, the acidity in the intracellular fluids damages cell nuclei, which controls cellular growth." [4]

"An acidic condition inhibits nerve action and an alkaline condition stimulates nerve action. One who has an alkaline blood condition can think and act (decide) well…. Therefore, it is very important to maintain an alkaline blood condition all the time—not only for physical health but also for mental awareness." [5]

Other Contributors

Dr. Robert M. Moldwin, MD, in his book *The Interstitial Cystitis Survival Guide* discusses the many problems that may account for the symptoms associated with IC. He states that a decrease of blood flow to the bladder wall could directly affect the nerves of the bladder leading to hypersensitivity and inflammation.

"Doctors Irwin and Galloway (1993) were the first to report a relative lack of blood flow in the bladders' of IC patients when compared to non-IC patients during bladder filling." [6]

An alkali-forming diet supplies the needed elements potassium, calcium, magnesium, sodium, and iron to help balance and maintain the body's pH. By maintaining a higher blood pH, one will decrease the body's acidity and increase alkalinity and body tissue perfusion with nutrients and oxygen. An alkali-forming diet/lifestyle eliminates the need for the body to try to store excess acid in the body's tissues to maintain its proper slightly high blood pH.

[1] Otto Warburg, *The Metabolism of Tumors*. London, England: Constabel, 1930

[2] Keichi Morishita, MD, *The Hidden Truth of Cancer*. San Francisco: George Ohsawa Macrobiotic Foundation, 1972

[3] Aihara, *Op. Cit.,* p. 111

[4] *Ibid.*, p. 112

[5] *Ibid.*, p. 109

[6] Dr. Robert M. Moldwin, MD, *The Interstitial Cystitis Survival Guide*, Oakland: New Harbinger Publications, 2000, p. 37

ANATOMY OF THE BLADDER

"If I'd known I was going to live so long, I'd have taken better care of myself."

— Leon Eldred

The urinary bladder is a temporary storage pouch for urine. It is composed of collapsible muscle and is located in front of the uterus and behind the pubic bone. The lower portion, continuous with the urethra, is called the neck; its upper tip, connected to the naval by a ligament, is called the apex.

The region between the two openings of the two ureters and the urethra is the trigone. The trigone area is the area that signals us to urinate. The muscles consist of interlacing smooth muscle fibers.

As the bladder fills with urine, it rises into the abdomen. Under normal conditions, the bladder can distend to hold 750ml to 1000ml (approximately one quart) of urine. When the bladder contains about 250ml (about one cup) of urine, the individual has a conscious desire to urinate. A moderately full bladder holds about 470ml (about two cups) of urine.

Two sphincters control the release of urine. The urethra is the end portion of the urinary system. A small tube carries urine by peristalsis from the bladder out of its urinary opening called the urinary meatus.

In women, the urethra is approximately 1½ inches long and is just above the opening of the vagina. Inside the urethra and the bladder is a lining called urothelial cells. This lining is protected by a mucous layer that keeps the tissue from being burned by acidic urine. This mucous layer is called the GAG layer (sulfated glycosaminoglycan). This GAG layer protects against acids and toxic elements.

In persons with interstitial cystitis, the GAG layer is compromised making the individual more susceptible to bacterial infections, toxins, and acidic urine.

CURRENT MEDICAL TREATMENTS

"To keep the body in good health is a duty... otherwise we shall not be able to keep the mind strong and clear."

— Gautama Buddha

I will briefly mention some current treatments for IC used in traditional allopathic medicine and do not intend to cover them thoroughly. There are numerous treatments currently for IC with most of the focus on the bladder per se. Since my resolution was a holistic approach, I will not cover in detail current urologic interventions, but will mention them in passing.

Hydrodistension is a treatment whereby the bladder is distended under anesthesia with sterile fluid for three hours. Some patients report being symptom-free for up to 6 months after this treatment. Intavesical therapy has been one of the cornerstones of treatment.

Silver nitrate, DMSO, and Chlorpactin are drugs that have been used intravesically (instilled into the bladder) with varying satisfactory responses with follow-ups of 6 to 24 months.

Some oral medications such as the following have been prescribed: antihistamines, muscle relaxants, narcotic pain meds, steroids, and antidepressants.

For further information on current medical treatments for IC, Dr. Moldwin's book *The Interstitial Cystitis Survival Guide* is a good reference.

Understanding Acid-Alkali Balance and its Effect on Interstitial Cystitis

"Just about every condition I can think of, from arthritis to diabetes to cancer, is associated with acidity. It is no coincidence that many of our modern habits such as alcohol consumption, smoking, eating sugar, and stress, all tend to increase acidity. The only parts of our body that are supposed to be acidic are the contents of the stomach, the skin, and perspiration. Virtually everything else is supposed to be at least slightly alkaline."

— Attributed to Dr. Robert C. Atkins, MD

Introduction

The majority of people in our American society today suffer from over acidity of the body's fluids that make up 70% of the body's weight. An interesting fact to note is that both our bodies and the earth are approximately 70% water. It is also known that our bodily fluids are related to the sea. The pH of seawater is approximately 7.8 while that of human blood is 7.4. This very sea inside each one of us is known as plasma, lymph, and cellular fluids that resemble the chemical composition of seawater. This "inner sea" circulates throughout our bodies, carrying life to every cell.

The maintenance of robust health comes from natural foods, oxygen, and pure water. The water in the body could be likened to swimming pool water. Swimming pools are strictly monitored at a certain pH level. The water should not be too acidic or too alkalotic. In IC, our body's pool of water has become too acidic.

"One school of thought says...disease is caused by germs

or some form of static disease-causing microbe (the germ theory)... Kill whatever is making you sick. [Treat the disease with] drugs, antibiotics, chemotherapy, radiation, [or] surgery.

"The other school of thought says most disease is caused by some imbalance in the body brought about by some nutritional, electrical, structural, toxicological or biological equation. In order to get well, you need to re-establish balance in your body.

"Embracing the biological view gives new insights to the disease process and is truly another paradigm for understanding health.

"Acids are a normal by-product of metabolism. The body has the mechanisms in place to eliminate these acids. But poor dietary habits, prolonged stress, lack of exercise, and toxicity exposures can lead to liver and kidney malfunction, and the acids in the body do not always get eliminated as they should.

"When the body has an excess of acid it can't get rid of, it gets stored for later removal. Where [is this acid stored]? In the interstitial spaces, also called the extracellular matrix - the spaces around the cells; the mesenchyme. When the body stores...(the acid) in the extracellular matrix, it believes that one day the acid is going to be removed. Therefore, in order to be in balance, it knows that for every molecule of acid that gets stored in the tissues, an equal molecule of bicarb or base needs to be put into the blood because one day it will need to escort the acid out of the body. If the body has an acid overload, it stores the acid in the tissues (the tissue pH decreases) and the blood compensates and becomes alkaline (the blood pH increases).

"The total healing of chronic illness only takes place when and if the blood is restored to a slightly alkaline pH. Normally, human blood stays in a very narrow pH range...around 7.3.

Below or above this range means symptoms and disease.

"When pH is too high or low, microorganisms in the blood can change shape, mutate, become pathogenic, and thrive. When [there is a] pH [imbalance]...enzymes that are constructive can become destructive[, and] oxygen delivery to cells suffer[s].

"Minerals have different pH levels at which they can be assimilated into the body. Minerals on the lower end of the atomic scale can be assimilated in a wider pH range, and minerals higher up on the scale require a narrower and narrower pH range in order to be assimilated by the body. For example, as more acid accumulates in our body, it gets stored and pushed further, and ultimately it gets pushed into the cell. When it gets pushed into the cell, the first thing it does is displace potassium and then magnesium and then sodium.

"Those are three critical minerals in our body. The potassium and magnesium will leave the body, but as a preservation mechanism the sodium will be retained. Remember, the body knows it must place an alkaline molecule in the blood to escort out this increasing acid that is being stored in the tissues and cells. What it will often do (when mineral reserves are low which is often the case when eating a modern American diet) is draw calcium (the most alkaline mineral known) from the bones and put it into the blood. This leads to something called free calcium excess.

"This is something you don't want and it is what's behind osteoporosis, arthritic pain, etc. It is brought about by the body compensating for an ever-increasing tissue acidosis somewhere in the body. What you don't want to do in this case is take more calcium supplements. With that said, you can now understand why calcium is one of the most over-prescribed supplements. In these situations what the body really needs is more potassium, and magnesium, perhaps organic sodium, and possibly zinc which lends help to the whole proper acid breakdown process." [1]

In order to understand how an alkali-forming diet/ lifestyle can help manage IC we will need to understand acid-alkali balance, pH, and some simple chemistry principles.

Defining pH

Briefly, we need to review some basic facts about acid-alkali balance to understand the chemical processes of the body. An acidic or alkaline substance is measured with a pH scale. pH stands for "potential of hydrogen." pH measures the amount of concentration of hydrogen ions in a solution. Hydrogen ions are acids that must be maintained within strict limits in the body. A high concentration of hydrogen ions means a solution is acidic. A low number of hydrogen ions mean the solution is alkaline. The pH scale is logarithmic, which means a difference of one pH unit represents a ten-fold increase or decrease in the concentration of hydrogen ions.

The pH scale, which determines whether something is acidic or alkaline, is numbered from 0 to 14. The pH of a solution is a measure of the number of hydrogen ions. The pH of a solution can range between 0 and 14. A neutral solution has a pH of 7. That is, there are an equal number of hydrogen ions (H^+) and hydroxide ions (OH^-). Solutions less than 7 are considered acidic and have a greater concentration of H^+. Solutions with a pH greater than 7 are basic or alkaline and have a greater concentration of OH^-.

Some examples of acid solutions are vinegar with a pH of 2.8 and coffee with a pH of 5.0. Arterial blood with a pH of 7.35 to 7.45 is alkaline. Blood needs to be slightly alkaline. A variation of 0.4 in either direction in the pH of the blood can be fatal. A pH less than 7.35 indicates a state of acidosis. A pH greater than 7.45 indicates a state of alkalosis.

A pH of 7 means the solution is neutral; it is a combination of acid and alkali together to create a neutral solution. Pure distilled water has a pH of 7. Pure distilled water is not acidic or alkaline; it is considered neutral. Baking soda, the household name for sodium bicarbonate, is an alkaline substance with a pH value of 8.3. Household ammonia is a strong alkali with a pH of 11. Remember, anything with a pH less than 7 is an acid and anything with a pH value greater than 7 is an alkali or base.

There are a number of body systems that have their preferred pH, as presented in Table 2. Examples are stomach acid with a pH of 1.0 or pancreatic fluids with a pH of 8.8. Urine pH is 4.6 to 8.0. Arterial blood has a pH of 7.4. Overall, the body's internal chemistry changes from a weak acid to a weak alkali within a 24-hour period, usually more acidic at dawn and more alkaline at sunset.

When the urine pH is in its normal range of 6.5 to 7.0, the blood pH is normal. A pH less than 6.0 is unhealthy (too acidic) and a pH greater than 8.5 is unhealthy (too alkaline.) When urine pH is 6.0 and below it indicates the body is ridding itself of excess H+ ions or acid, and it indicates the body is in an acidic state.

The urine pH in the **bladder** of persons with IC has been reported by Dr. Gillespie to be on the alkaline side. However, she also reports the urine samples of the IC patients taken with a catheter from their **kidneys** was acidic. The following excerpt from Dr. Lark reads as follows regarding the urine pH of persons with IC.

"To test for interstitial cystitis, a urine sample is normally analyzed for the presence of bacteria. The urine should show no sign of bacterial infection and often has an alkaline pH. As mentioned above, when bladder cells are damaged, they become more acidic. They leak their contents into the urine, losing

Table 1: pH Values for Common Substances

Substance	pH Value	State
Hydrochloric Acid, (Drain Cleaner)	0.1	Acid
Sulfuric Acid (Battery Acid)	0.3	
Cola	2.5	
Vinegar (5% Acetic Acid)	2.8	
Wine	2.8 - 3.8	
Lemon Juice (Citric Acid)	3.0	
Orange Juice	3.0	
Apples	3.0	
Tomato Juice	4.0	
Black Coffee	5.0	
Detergent	6.5	
Milk	6.8	
Distilled Water	7.0	Neutral
Seawater	7.8	Alkali
Baking Soda	8.3	
Milk of Magnesia	10.7	
Household Bleach	11.0	
Household Ammonia	11.0	
Caustic Soda (Drain Cleaner)	14.0	

Table 2: pH Values for Bodily Substances

Substance	pH Value
Stomach Acid	1.0
Skin	4.5 - 6.0
Urine	4.6 - 8.0
Saliva	5.0 - 7.5
Breast Milk	6.6 - 6.9
Perspiration	7.0 - 8.0
Tears	7.2
Arterial Blood	7.4
Intestinal Fluid	7.7
Bile	8.0
Pancreatic Fluid	8.8

their alkaline minerals while, at the same time, gaining acidic hydrogen ions from the surrounding environment. Thus the cells become more acidic while the urine pH begins to rise. The overacidity of the cells makes it more difficult for the bladder tissue to repair itself." [2]

In my case, my urine pH was very acidic around 4.6 because of my high acid-forming diet. If you find in testing your urine pH your urine is more on the alkaline side you will understand the dynamics of eating an acid-forming diet and still coming up with an alkaline urine. It is not so important that you measure your urine pH. Measure the pH of your saliva instead. This will give you an even better indication where your body's pH lies. See the chapter "How to Measure your pH" for details on measuring pH.

Buffer Systems

We need to understand that in the process of living and daily activities as well as digesting our food our bodies produce acids. Our body's movements and exercise produce acids such as lactic acid and carbon dioxide. In water, carbon dioxide becomes carbonic acid. Phosphoric and sulfuric acids are produced from the metabolism of proteins and grains. These acids must be buffered and eliminated from the body. "This acid load can be divided into two major components: **volatile acid** and **nonvolatile acid**.

1. Volatile Acid. This is carbonic acid (H_2CO_3) which can be readily converted to a gas (CO_2) and water and vice versa.

$$H_2CO_3 <\!\!-\!\!> CO_2 + H_2O$$

2. Nonvolatile Acid. Nonvolatile acids cannot be converted to gases under physiological circumstances. In western countries, where much protein (often in the form of meat) is consumed, about 40-100 mmol of nonvolatile (or noncarbonic) acid are produced by metabolism each day. The most important nonvolatile acid is sulfuric acid. It is produced from the metabolism of sulfur-containing amino acids and accounts for about 75% of the nonvolatile acid. Phosphoric acid is produced from the metabolism of nucleic acids and phospholipids. It is a minor component of the nonvolatile acid produced, but becomes an important buffer in the renal excretion of acid (see below). Lactic acid accumulates during exercise.

Alkali. Although most people have a net production of nonvolatile acid, they also produce alkali from the ingestion of milk, fruit, and vegetables. This production of alkali results from the metabolism of the salts of weak organic acids (e.g., sodium or potassium lactate, citrate, and isocitrate) contained in these foods. Remember, these are the salts of the weak organic acids, not the acids themselves, that are ingested. Metabolism of these salts consumes H+ ions. The H+ comes from H_2CO_3 leaving increased amounts of HCO_3- in the blood. Strict vegetarians may eat sufficient fruits and vegetables that they have a net production of alkali, rather than a net production of nonvolatile acid (although they will still produce nonvolatile acid)." [3]

The body buffers and eliminates acids to maintain its acid-alkali balance. An example of buffering is taking an antacid for heartburn. There are three main buffering systems: the lungs, the kidneys, and blood buffers. These systems keep the body from becoming too acidic or too alkaline. If for some reason these organ-buffering systems weaken, the body's pH balance will be upset. Either too much or too little acid will be neutralized.

The lungs exhale CO_2 or carbon dioxide—an acid waste from metabolism—and inhale O_2 or oxygen—an alkaline element that is diffused into the blood stream.

The kidneys can generate, retain, or excrete bicarbonate ions (alkali) or hydrogen ions (acid) thereby increasing or decreasing the body's pH.

Blood buffers are the bicarbonate/carbonic acid system,

the phosphates, proteins, and hemoglobin buffer systems. The bicarbonate/carbonic acid system is the most important. This buffer system is immediate and continuous in contributing or accepting hydrogen ion concentration thereby regulating the blood's pH.

The blood stream is the most critically buffered system of the entire body. Arterial and venous blood must maintain a slightly alkaline pH: arterial blood pH is 7.4, but venous blood is 7.36 due to a higher level of carbonic acid. The pH of interstitial fluids and connective tissue—body tissues, organs, and joints—is 7.34 to 7.36, a slightly more acidic profile, because cells dump as much acid as possible into these areas, buffering the blood.

Overly acidic cells lose their flexibility. In the case of red blood cells for example, the loss of flexibility inhibits the elasticity and adaptability of the cells, thus impeding blood flow.

Dr. Kern, the German heart specialist, was the first to discover that heart infarct is caused by over acidity. His research revealed that blood that flows through acid tissue itself becomes acidic. When the pH of the heart is at or below 6.4, the red blood cells become inflexible and unable to deform sufficiently to pass through the narrow capillaries. Once the red blood cells are attached against the capillary walls, they cause a blockage.

According to Dr. Kern, heart infarct is nothing more than a gigantic acid catastrophe. Dr. Moldwin in his book *The Interstitial Cystitis Survival Guide* reports, "Dr. Irwin and Galloway (1993) were the first to report a relative lack of blood flow in the bladders of IC patients when compared to non-IC patients during bladder filling." [4] I believe the lack of blood flow to the bladder is related to acid buildup around the tissues of the bladder, which causes the red blood cells to deform. As stated above by Dr. Kern, the capillaries are obstructed by these deformed red blood cells and cause decreased circulation to the bladder. Decreased circulation to the bladder will cause pain and inflammation.

Eating a highly acid-forming diet taxes the body's mineral buffering systems (potassium, calcium, sodium, and magnesium) and the blood pH is maintained slightly alkaline at the expense of the tissues, organs, and joints by dumping excess acids quickly into the cells and interstitial fluids. pH in these areas can drop dangerously to concentrations of pH equal to 5.0.

An example the reader may be familiar with of acid dumping into joints is the disease gout where a high protein diet is converted to uric acid in the body. The uric acid deposits settle in different joints, and are exacerbated by alcohol and a high protein diet. In IC, acid can be deposited in and around the interstitial tissues of the bladder and can damage the cellular oxygen respiration mechanism. The symptoms of pain, burning, and frequency are related to decreased oxygen to the nerves and tissues of the bladder. The GAG layer is diminished related to decreased circulation.

When buffering the body's acids in the bloodstream the following events occur: "The family of mineral compounds which neutralize acids are the carbonic salts, symbolized as $BaCO_3$ where the Ba stands for any one of the four base or alkaline elements. Na, Ca, K, Mg (sodium, calcium, potassium, magnesium.) When carbonic salts meet with strong acids such as sulfuric acid, phosphoric acid, acetic acid, and lactic acid, the alkaline minerals making up the carbonic salt leave the salt and combine with the acids to make new salts. For example:

$$BaCO_3 + H_2SO_4 = BaSO_4 + H_2O + CO_2$$

Carbonic Salt + Sulfuric Acid
= Sulfuric Salt + Water + Carbon Dioxide

In the result, carbonic salt changes sulfuric acid, which is a strong acid, to sulfuric salt, which can be eliminated through the kidneys without any harm. In the same way, some other acid may be changed to another salt and be eliminated through the wall of the large intestine. In short, the acids, which are the product of metabolism, can be eliminated only after they are changed to neutral salts. Then they are no longer harmful to the kidneys and to the wall of the intestine.

The result of this change, that is to say, from acid to neutral salt is to reduce the concentration of alkaline elements such as Na, Ca, Mg, and K in the blood and then in the extracellular fluid. It is the lowered concentration of alkaline elements, which is referred to as the acidic condition of the body fluid. Since in order for us to be healthy our body fluid must be kept at an alkaline level (pH of 7.4) we must re-supply the lost alkaline elements through the foods we eat." [5]

The need to convert aggressive acids into salts robs contemporary man of essential minerals and trace minerals.

For example, if our diets are deficient in the alkaline elements (Na, Ca, K, Mg), the body will strip calcium from bone or arterial walls in order to render phosphoric acid harmless by converting it into a salt. This is the cause of such diseases as osteoporosis and the so-called "hardening of the arteries."

In metabolic acidosis—a disturbance of the body acid-alkali balance in which there is excessive acidity of body fluids or loss of alkali—, K+ (potassium) inside the cell exchanges for excess acid or H+ (hydrogen) across the cell membranes and then K+ is excreted. Over time, the K+ stores inside the body's cells become depleted and the cell becomes more acidic. This is how our body tissues and organs begin to become gradually more acidic over time.

Lifestyle

§ Many aspects of modern life promote over acidity. Some contributors to over acidity are:

§ Diet with excess of foods such as proteins, starches, sugar, salt, sodas, caffeine, alcohol, and refined and processed foods, which deplete ones alkaline minerals

§ Drinking acid water

§ Inhaling polluted acidic air

§ Diet deficient of the foods that help neutralize acid such as fresh fruits, vegetables and dairy

§ Sedentary life styles

§ Too much stress with inadequate rest and relaxation

§ Exposure to toxic chemicals in our environment and personal care

§ Consuming foods grown in mineral and nutrient depleted topsoil

§ Shallow breathing limiting our inhalation of alkalizing oxygen and retaining acidic carbon dioxide instead of fully exhaling it

§ Eating on the go, neglecting to relax and chew adequately allowing the alkaline salivary glands in the mouth to start digestion

Allergies

It has been suggested that the etiology of allergies starts because the body is in such an acidic state. With allergies, you have inflammation and cell destruction related to the inflammation. This contributes to an acidic state and thus creates a vicious cycle. Potassium has proved effective in treating allergies.

Minerals

There are mineral imbalances and nutrition deficiencies that develop after years of a high acid-forming diet and insufficient intake of the buffering alkali-forming foods.

When the body becomes overly acidic some of the following symptoms can develop: food allergies, low energy, muscular pain and fatigue, heartburn, lack of sex drive, joint pain, inflammatory conditions, cystitis, uretheritis, urinary infection, memory loss, etc.

The Aging Process

The organs in the body decline in function by approximately one percent per year after the age of forty and faster in some cases depending on the person's diet, stress level, exposure to pollutants, and general life style. As we age, the slightly alkaline balance in our cells and tissues declines. As our cells and tissues become more acidic over time, the ability to deliver nutrients and oxygen to the cells declines. An example of acid buildup and decreased blood flow is when your leg "falls asleep." Blood flow is decreased allowing acid buildup. The leg has a funny "pins and needles" feeling most of us have experienced. Upon standing, blood flow is restored. The tingly pins and needles sensation subsides.

Diet

Most Americans are eating an inverted diet of 80% *acid-forming* foods and only 20% *alkali-forming* foods. Acid-forming foods are high in sulfur, phosphorus, and chlorine. These foods include high protein foods, meat, grains, acidic water, and soft drinks. Additionally, coffee, alcoholic drinks, sugar, and salt are all acid-forming.

"As the pH of the blood goes more acid, fatty acids which are normally electro-magnetically charged on the negative side switch to positive and automatically are attracted to and begin to stick to the walls of arteries which are electro-magnetically charged on the negative side. (And as science states, opposites attract.) It should start to make sense that a society which over-emphasizes food that could push blood more acid will have a high rate of heart disease." [6]

Alkali-forming foods are rich in potassium, calcium, magnesium, iron, and sodium. These foods include fruits, vegetables, and dairy.

"In fruit and most vegetables, the organic acid (such as the acidity of an orange which you can taste) contains many elements such as potassium, calcium, and magnesium. Organic acids, when oxidized, become carbon dioxide and water; the alkaline elements (K, Na, Ca, Mg) remain and neutralize body acid. In other words, strangely enough, acid foods reduce body acids. This is the reason that fruits and most vegetables are considered alkaline forming foods. Conversely, high protein foods and most grains, when metabolized, produce acid that must be neutralized; therefore they are generally acid forming foods." [7]

The body's alkaline reserves help to buffer and neutralize metabolic acids. Ninety-eight percent of the body's alkaline element *potassium* is found inside our cells. Ninety-nine percent of *calcium* is found in bones and teeth, while seventy percent of *magnesium* is found in the bones. Forty percent of *sodium* is found in bone and fifty percent is found in the extracellular fluid. The major proportion of *iron* in the body is found in the blood in the form of hemoglobin. I will address these alkaline elements later in more detail in the chapter "Starting an Alkalizing Program."

Alkalinity and Mental Health

"The effect of pH on mental health is well demonstrated in the work of Dr. William H. Philpott, MD, an environmental psychiatrist who spent many years researching the links between food allergies, overacidity, and mood. In treating mental illness over a twenty-five year period, he frequently observed that these conditions were often not emotional in origin but rather were due to chemical imbalances." [8]

"One physiological reason for the link between alkalinity and optimism is that overacidity acts as a depressant to the central nervous system, whereas alkalinity acts as a natural mood elevator. When acids accumulate in tissues throughout the body, they can directly affect the mental energy underlying our ability to create and maintain a positive outlook..." [9]

Summary

To summarize, what has been explained thus far is that as one ages an acid-alkali imbalance develops and we live in a state of over acidity of the body's cells and tissues. What causes this over acidity can be attributed to many factors including the aging process and decreased function of the organs that help eliminate acids, a high acid-forming diet, a stressful life style, breathing polluted air, poor intake of buffering alkali-forming foods like fruits, vegetables and dairy, consuming acidic water, colas, coffee, alcohol, and shallow breathing. Medications and many over the counter meds are acidifying including ibuprofen, aspirin, and even nutritional vitamin C is acidic. Our body needs to maintain a blood pH of 7.35 to 7.45 and needs to neutralize and eliminate acids at all costs, even if that means dumping acids inside and around our cells, tissues and organs. In the case of IC, these acids are being dumped into the interstitial tissues around the bladder. These acid wastes around the bladder tissue may cause the deformity of the red blood cells flowing through acid tissues. These red blood cells deform and occlude the capillary flow of blood to the bladder.

The lack of blood flow causes a decrease of nutrients and oxygen to the bladder and nerves. When the pH is too low, the oxygen delivery to our cells suffers. With decreased oxygen and decreased blood flow, you experience pain.

Essentially, what is happening in the body can be explained using simple chemistry. Life and the process of metabolism create an acid load in the body that must be neutralized or buffered by an intake of alkaline foods and drinks. In other words, we are attempting to combine an acid (body metabolism) and an alkali (alkali-forming diet/lifestyle) in approximately equal amounts in order to maintain a neutral or balanced state in our bodies. By working to establish this balanced state, we will maintain our blood, tissues, organs, and cells in a slightly alkaline condition, which will provide the healthy environment we need to thrive. Neutrality is an ideal condition in which the amount of acid and alkali is equal. It is an ideal condition and not realistic. However, in reality, our diet and lifestyle choices are typically more acidic or alkaline.

[1] http://www.cfsdoc.org/biological_terrain.htm

[2] Lark, *Op. Cit.*, pp 84-85

[3] Dr. Dantzler, http://human.physiol.arizona.edu/sched/renal/dant49/Dantzler.L49.html , Body Buffers

[4] Moldwin, Op. Cit., p. 37

[5] Aihara, Op. Cit., pp. 9 - 10

[6] Dr. William Philpott, MD, *Biomagnetic Handbook*, Enviro-Tech Products, 1989

[7] Aihara, *Op. Cit.*, p. 23.

[8] Lark, *Op. Cit.*, p. 67

[9] Ibid., p. 68

HOW TO MEASURE YOUR BODY'S pH

"Unless the doctors of today become the dietitians of tomorrow, the dietitians of today will become the doctors of tomorrow."

— Dr. Alexis Carrel, *Man the Unknown* (1935)

Urine pH

Normally, urine is slightly acidic especially in the morning because the body produces acids in the metabolic processes that occur continuously in the body. In a *healthy pH-balanced* body, urine is slightly acidic in the morning (pH is 6.5 to 7.0) generally becoming more alkaline (pH is 7.5 to 8.0) by evening as the body digests food and releases alkali elements. A person consuming an acid-forming diet will generally have a urine pH below 6 indicating the body is attempting to eliminate excess acid.

Table 3: Urine pH States

Unhealthy (Acidic)	Healthy	Unealthy (Alkaline)
< 6	7 - 8	> 8

You can purchase a roll of pH paper usually sold at pharmacies to measure the saliva and urine pH. There is a color chart included with the roll of pH paper. Yellow indicates acid and blue, alkali.

When checking your urine, collect fresh urine in a clean dry container. Remove a strip from the pH paper or strip (do not touch the strip area itself that is to be dipped) and completely immerse in fresh urine and remove immediately to avoid dissolving out reagents. While removing the strip from the urine specimen, run the edge of the strip on the rim of the container to remove excess urine. Hold the strip in a horizontal position and compare the strip to the corresponding color chart. Hold the strip close to the color blocks and match carefully. pH may be read up to one minute after dipping.

Urine pH ranges from 4.6 to 8, however urine pH below 6 usually indicates an overly acidic state in the body. Maintaining my urine pH close to 7 made me feel the best.

Saliva pH

To check the saliva, wait at least 2 hours after eating or drinking. Fill your mouth with saliva and then swallow it. Do this again to help ensure that the saliva is clean. Then the third time, put some saliva onto pH paper.

The pH paper should turn blue. This indicates that your saliva is slightly alkaline at a healthy pH of 7.4. If it is not blue, compare the color with the chart that comes with the pH paper.

"When healthy, the pH of blood is 7.4, the pH of spinal fluid is 7.4, and the pH of saliva is 7.4. Thus the pH of saliva parallels the extra cellular fluid...pH test of saliva represents the most consistent and most definitive physical sign of the ionic calcium deficiency syndrome...The pH of the non-deficient and healthy person is in the 7.5 (dark blue) to 7.1 (blue) slightly alkaline range. The range from 6.5 (blue-green) which is weakly acidic to 4.5 (light yellow) which is strongly acidic represents states from mildly deficient to strongly deficient, respectively. Most children are dark blue, a pH of 7.5. Over half of adults are green-yellow, a pH of 6.5 or lower, reflecting the calcium deficiency of aging and lifestyle defects. Cancer patients are usually a bright yellow, a pH of 4.5, especially when terminal." [1]

One should check the saliva or urine the same time every day preferably in the mornings when one awakens to determine the trend of the body's pH. One should check them over a period of weeks to months to evaluate the body's pH trend.

[1] Robert R. Barefoot and Carl J. Reich, MD, *The Calcium Factor: The Scientific Secret of Health and Youth*, Arkansas City, Kansas: Gilliland Printing Inc., 1996.

LEAKY GUT SYNDROME

"If we could give every individual the right amount of nourishment and exercise, not too little and not too much, we would have found the safest way to health."

— Hippocrates c. 460 - 377 BC

Leaky gut syndrome or LGS needs to be addressed in persons with IC since it also contributes to the food allergies and inflammation experienced by so many persons with IC. Food allergies and inflammation contribute to the body's acidity. In addition, food allergies can manifest as bladder pain and inflammation. LGS is a condition where the small intestine becomes inflamed and large spaces develop between the cells of the gut wall creating excessive permeability. A healthy intact small intestine is normally designed to be selectively permeable to very tiny microscopic food particles and nutrients.

However, with LGS, undesirable agents cross into the bloodstream such as disease-causing bacteria (salmonella etc.), yeasts (Candida), *large allergenic food molecules*, toxins, and chemicals, e.g., food additives. Malabsorption and malnutrition can occur at the same time. Many nutrients have to be actively transported across the gut wall and these active carrying sites can be damaged in the intestines leading to nutritional deficiency.

The following conditions are just some of the problems that can develop with LGS: *food allergies*, eczema, asthma, migraine, chronic fatigue syndrome, autoimmune diseases, arthritis, lupus, multiple sclerosis, irritable bowel syndrome, and *inflammatory conditions* in general.

What causes the LGS?

   Antibiotics, which wipe out friendly gut bacteria, allow yeast and disease-causing bacteria to flourish. These yeast and parasitic bacteria damage the gut wall and can enter the blood stream causing disease in other parts of the body.

   Nonsteroidal anti-inflammatory drugs (NSAIDS) like aspirin and ibuprofen can irritate and damage the gut wall.

   Alcohol and caffeine are strong gut irritants.

   In addition, when we are under stress (having a chronic condition like IC is a big stressor) and we are in a fight or flight mode, there is decreased blood circulation to the gastrointestinal tract. If you have been storing up stress response for a long time, your intestinal tract will be chronically "starved" for blood and will start to function imperfectly.

   When the gut is leaky it allows large food particles to enter the blood stream, the body sees these large food particles as foreign bodies that must be combated with an immune response. This causes an inflammatory response (histamine), and thus a food allergy is born.

Clear®

In order to begin my own healing process with LGS I discovered an herbal course of treatment called Clear®. It is a 600-year-old herbal recipe from the East, an extremely effective yeast-parasite cleansing formula that effectively kills all macro and micro parasites and strengthens the intestines. Clear® also has strong antifungal properties and is effective against Candida albicans.

The Awareness Corporation that sells these herbs

recommends taking Clear® with two other herbal formulas called Experience™, which is supposed to tonify the bowel, and Harmony™, which nourishes and rebuilds. As of this writing, I have personally only used the Clear® formula with excellent results. My energy level has improved immensely—since the yeast and "bad" bacteria are not consuming all my nutrients—, and my allergies are improving.

Probiotics

In addition, to help repair the bowels probiotics are vital to replenish the good bacteria that are destroyed with the use of antibiotics. The following are some protective and therapeutic roles probiotics perform in the intestinal tract:

§ Kill and deactivate hostile and disease causing bacteria;

§ Detoxify pollutants and carcinogens;

§ Improve the efficiency of the digestive tract;

§ Eliminate constipation, diarrhea;

§ Manufacture certain B vitamins;

§ Manufacture milk-digesting enzymes that help digest calcium-rich dairy products

It is recommended to take good quality freeze-dried bacteria such as Lactobacillus acidophilus or Lactobacillus bulgaricus. Good supplements are found in the refrigerated section of a health food store and manufactured with a filtration process.

Probiotics should not be taken with food to avoid extreme acidity during mealtimes. In addition, take EC or enteric-coated probiotics, which will allow the capsule to be digested in the intestines where it is needed—not the stomach. Good products should carry a guarantee of viable colonizing bacteria up to a specific date. Probiotics should be used

§ During and after antibiotic therapy;

§ By peri- and post-menopausal women to reduce chances of osteoporosis;

§ By anyone having recurrent bladder and vaginal infections;

§ By anyone with chronic health problems

ALLERGIES

"One Man's Meat is Another Man's Poison"

—Lucretius

A person can be allergic to anything: food or beverages, chemicals, pollen and natural environmental allergies, animals, et cetera. According to Dr. Moldwin[1], 40.6% of persons with IC also have allergies to something. A history of antibiotics predisposes one to LGS and its related allergies. Dr. Devi S. Nambudripad, DC, LAc, RN, PhD, author of *Say Goodbye to Illness* states, "An allergy is an adverse physical, physiological, and/or psychological response of an individual towards one or more substances also known as allergens." [2]

The literal meaning of allergy comes from the Greek word *allos* or "altered action." A person has a biological hypersensitivity to certain substances. Traditional allergists describe an allergy as an attack of a person's own body when it comes in contact with an allergen and reacts adversely even though that substance may actually be harmless to the body. The reaction of the person's immune system towards the allergen produces IgE antibodies and IgG antibodies that release histamines that produce the different allergic reactions such as sneezing, coughing, itchy and watery eyes, sinusitis, headaches, anxiety, hyperactivity especially in children (ADHD), all kinds of inflammatory conditions or in the case of IC inflammation and burning of the bladder tissue when exposed to the allergen. The most common sites that are affected by allergic reactions are skin, eye, nose, throat, mouth, rectum, and vaginal mucosa.

Pain in the vulva or Vulvodynia is seen in approximately 10% of persons with IC and may be explained by possibly two causes once infection or skin diseases have been ruled out:

1. That it may be a manifestation of an allergic reaction and/or

2. A manifestation of decreased circulation of oxygen and nutrients related to hyperacidity surrounding the nerves and tissues of the vulva related to an overly acidic diet/lifestyle.

Dr. Lark states the severity of allergic reactions depends on the degree of acidity of the internal environment of the body. "When the body is overly acidic, and mast cells are activated by an allergen, they will tend to break down more quickly and are more likely to generate histamines and other inflammatory chemicals. Overacidity can both trigger the symptoms of and lengthen the period of convalescence in allergic individuals. Unfortunately, the underlying cause is often over-acidity, which is rarely treated. Many people are unaware of the role that overacidity plays in the reactivity to allergens." [3] Of course, one should avoid the offending allergens, but the key is to start an alkalizing program.

Foods that commonly cause allergies are as follows: wheat, dairy, rye, corn, soy, chocolate, tomatoes, strawberries, nuts, shellfish, eggs, pork.

"Safe" or commonly hypo-allergenic foods that one may wish to start an alkalizing program with are the following: parsnips, turnips, rutabaga, sweet potatoes, yams, celery, zucchini, carrots, peaches, pears, trout, cod and mackerel.

Elimination and rotation diets and homeopathy will be briefly defined as follows:

Elimination Diet: was developed by Dr. Albert H. Rowe and must be followed for a period to determine which foods are responsible for the allergic symptoms. If a fruit allergy is suspected, for example, all fruits are eliminated until symptoms subside and foods are added one at a time until a normal diet is attained.

Rotation Diet: a different group of food is eaten every day for a week. In this method, seven groups of food are eaten each day of the week with something different each day. This way, reactions to any group can be traced and eliminated.

Homeopathy: In this treatment minute concentration of the offending foods is used to prepare sublingual drops. Homeopathy is like a vaccine where the body is exposed to a dilute amount of the allergen and then builds up a resistance to the offending allergen after exposure to it in this diluted form.

Food allergies can be detected by blood testing for IgG and IgE antibodies. An allergist who is a medical doctor can order blood tests to determine allergies. Other professional health care providers such as naturopaths, homeopaths, and osteopaths can order blood tests through the mail.

If you are interested in testing yourself the needleless way at home there is a simple pain-free procedure called Muscle Response Testing (MRT.) Biokinesiology (MRT) was discovered by a chiropractor Dr. George Goodheart, in the 1960's. He found that certain muscles were weak or strong muscles became weak when he touched certain acupuncture points on the body. He was able to determine organic imbalances in the person. Later he related these differences to foods and food supplements that would strengthen weak muscles and tonify the individual.

In her book, Dr. Nambudripad describes the procedure MRT: "Muscle Response Testing is the body's communication pathway with the brain. Through MRT, the patient can be tested for various allergens. MRT is a standard test used in applied kinesiology to compare the strength of a predetermined test muscle in the presence and absence of a suspected allergen. If the particular muscle (test muscle) weakens in the presence of an item, it signifies that the item is an allergen. If the muscle remains strong, the substance is not an allergen." [4]

In a pilot study attempted to determine the efficiency of MRT in detecting food allergies, the serum test for IgE and IgG confirmed 19 of 21 food allergies that tested positive (muscle weakening or inhibition) with MRT having a screening efficiency rate of 90.5%.

Regarding MRT, simply stated, the human body is generally an efficient electrical current and when it comes in contact with an allergen this allergen "short-circuits" our system and causes a weakness in the current (muscle weakness when tested with MRT.)

MRT Technique: [5] There is an examiner and an examinee (the one being tested.) Stand about two feet apart from each other facing each others left or right shoulder; take care that you do not stand right in front of each other. You can choose either arm to begin with and you can alternate them when one arm tires out.

Let us say we will start with testing the examinee's left arm strength. You are about two feet apart from each other and you the examiner are looking at the examinee's left shoulder. Next, place your left palm firmly on the examinee's right shoulder to begin a circuit of energy flow. The examinee's arms are hanging loose at their sides and the examinee is looking straight ahead. Now have the examinee raise their left arm straight out approximately 90 degrees (it does not have to be exactly 90 degrees) in front or off to the side with the left hand hanging loose, slightly flexed downwardly. The examiner

MRT Technique

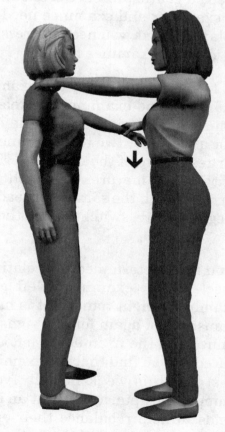

Examinee   **Examiner**

will press down with the right hand on the examinee's left wrist joint. (Examiner's skin touching the skin of the examinee's wrist.) You only need a gentle pressure of about 5 to 7 pounds of pressure. Both examiner and examinee need to keep their hands open and relaxed. Next, you need to press gently on the examinee's wrist while the examinee resists.

You are not trying to overpower the examinee; you are determining as examiner and examinee the relative strength of the indicator muscle of the examinee. The examiner will press downward for a second or two to determine the indicator muscle strength or resistance of the examinee. The examiner needs to press with the same pressure each time and the examinee needs to resist with the same effort each time. If you or the examinee begins to tire, switch to the other arm or take a break.

Now that you have determined the relative strength of the indicator muscle of the examinee's left arm place the allergen in the examinee's right hand that is hanging loosely at their side and muscle test again for any signs of weakening of the indicator muscle of the examinee's left arm when the allergen is introduced. If you find that the examinee's baseline indicator muscle strength is weak initially, you can gently massage the examinee's acupuncture point an inch under the navel for 30 seconds to help rebalance their energy and try retesting the muscle strength again before testing with an allergen.

Oval Ring Test: You can also test with an oval ring test. The examinee sits in a comfortable chair while pressing the ring finger and thumb together firmly while the examiner applies a gentle pressure to pull the fingers apart.

You can determine the indicator muscle strength of the examinee's finger grip and then introduce an allergen and test for any weakening. When the indicator ring finger gets tired, you can use the index and thumb or the middle finger and thumb then switch hands when the examinee gets tired. I prefer the oval ring test myself.

Oval Ring Test

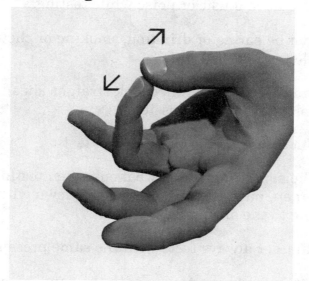

It will take some practice to determine the baseline strength of the muscles or grip being tested, but with practice, you can become very proficient at this MRT.

If you wish to test a surrogate such as a pet, infant or child, or invalid have the examinee hold the pet or infant/child. The child or invalid can touch the skin of the examinee while the examinee holds the allergen. You must maintain skin to skin contact of the examinee and surrogate otherwise the surrogate will not receive the results of the testing. The examiner's hand needs to touch the skin of the examinee respectively also.

If the examinee (or surrogate) is allergic to an allergen, the indicator muscle will weaken. If the examinee (or surrogate) is not allergic to the allergen, the muscle will remain strong.

Rules to Follow While Doing MRT

§ Avoid fluorescent lighting.

§ Remove jewelry.

§ Do not have music or noise while testing.

§ Do not be eating or drinking, smoking or chewing gum while testing.

§ Examiner and examinee look straight ahead and try to relax as much as possible.

§ Do not cross hands or feet when testing.

§ If the arm being tested weakens when testing an allergen, push the arm all the way down with a full swing to the examinee's side.

§ Examiner always tests with the same pressure.

§ Examinee always resists with the same pressure.

§ Be patient and practice the MRT technique for best results.

Finally, for those of you who are open-minded, curious, and wish to eliminate all of your allergies, Dr. Devi Nambudripad, has written a book *Say Goodbye to Illness*. [6] In her book, she discusses allergies and related health disorders and has established NAET (Nambudripad's Allergy Elimination Techniques) where she claims to combine allopathy, acupuncture, chiropractic, kinesiology, and nutrition to create a unique healing technique to permanently eliminate allergies. She states that over 2500 licensed medical practioners have been trained in NAET worldwide.

[1] Moldwin, *Op. Cit.*, p. 43

[2] Devi S. Nambudripad, DC, LAc, RN, PhD, (Acu), *Say Goodbye to Illness, 2nd Edition*, Buena Park: Delta Publishing Company, 1999, p. 9

[3] Lark, *Op. Cit.*, p. 75

[4] Nambudripad, *Op. Cit*, p.70

[5] Adapted from *Which Vitamin, Which Herb Do I Need, 3rd,* Shady Cove, OR: Biokenesiology Institute, 1984, pp. 17- 23

[6] Nambudripad, *Op. Cit.*

THE LIVER

"The sun, with all those planets revolving around it and dependent on it, can still ripen a bunch of grapes as if it had nothing else in the universe to do."

— Galileo

Most of us are routinely exposed to nicotine, toxins of various kinds and a whole host of synthetic drugs from ibuprofen to steroids.

Most of us overeat the wrong things and pass up what is good for us. High fat, high sugar, high protein diets stress the liver. Overeating especially overcooked, fatty foods puts added strain on the liver. LGS puts another stress on the liver. In addition, lack of exercise has an indirect effect on the liver. When we do not exercise, an excess of toxins can build up and has to be transformed by the liver.

Many of us eat diets that are too high in protein, take over-the-counter, or prescription drugs, and routinely expose ourselves to radiation and other pollutants. Everything we breath, eat and absorb through our skin is detoxified by the liver. Some of the more detrimental compounds we ingest that increase the liver's workload include:

§ High protein diets

§ Alcohol

§ Caffeine

§ Nicotine

- Pesticides and herbicides

- Saturated fats

- Heavy metals

Dr. Andrew Weil, MD, author of *Natural Health, Natural Medicine* says, "High protein diets impose a considerable work load on the digestive system and may contribute to feelings of fatigue and lack of energy."

According to the American Liver Foundation, liver diseases are the fourth leading cause of death up to the age of 65. It is not commonly known that a significant incidence of liver disease exists in this country. In the past, liver disease was only associated with chronic alcoholics. Now, however, liver disease strikes obese people, social drinkers, and people who eat poorly.

Responsibility of the Liver
The liver is responsible for detoxifying the body. Anytime we ingest potentially harmful chemicals, which include drugs or alcohol, liver cells must filter out these compounds.

Even if you do not suffer from any liver disease or do not abuse alcohol, you may still require liver cleansing. Everything that enters the liver through the portal vein must be detoxified and neutralized.

A poorly functioning liver can underlie chronic fatigue including Chronic Fatigue Syndrome (CFS) and allergies. Even if the liver has sustained only minimal damage, the immune system can be compromised

This effect has been observed in laboratory tests. For example, in some instances, liver injury has resulted in the rampant development of yeast infections throughout the body.

The liver plays an integral role in so many other body systems and organs. Anyone who suffers from compromised liver function will experience chronic fatigue in combination with other symptoms.

The liver also plays a role in stabilizing blood sugar levels, which can contribute to food cravings and appetite surges.

The Benefits of Milk Thistle

Milk thistle can help prevent the subtle kind of liver damage to which any of us may be susceptible. The flavonoids contained in milk thistle have a strong liver protective action and have been extensively used in Europe as pharmaceutical preparations for liver disorders.

The active ingredients in milk thistle consist of a complex of compounds, which are referred to as silymarin. These substances can actually protect the liver against certain toxins, while simultaneously boosting the function of the liver. Milk thistle contains some of the most potent liver-protecting substances known. For this reason, it is an invaluable herb for the treatment of hepatitis, cirrhosis, jaundice and fatty degeneration of the liver.

In addition, milk thistle can legitimately be called an antioxidant. It helps protect the cells from free radicals by scavenging them before they can cause cellular damage.

Milk thistle also acts to protect the kidneys, brain, and other vital organs from toxin damage, treats allergic reactions, reduces inflammation, and promotes healing. It also helps to emulsify fats and enhance bile flow, making it a good remedy for indigestion.

Most health food stores stock this herb under the name of milk thistle; however, it may also be found as Thisilyn, Silymarin, or Silybum.

[1] The information in this section has been adapted from www.nutraceutical.com/educate/pdf/milkthistle.pdf

GALLBLADDER / LIVER FLUSH

"For all things produced in a garden, whether of salads or fruits, a poor man will eat better that has one of his own, than a rich man that has none."

— J. C. Loudoun

Your liver keeps your blood clean while your gallbladder secretes bile necessary for digestion. Keeping these organs clean and healthy helps your entire system function better. A gallbladder/ liver flush is important to help increase the flow of alkaline bile (pH of 8) into the digestive tract. This flow of alkaline bile helps to neutralize the acid load in the body. Bile helps to break down fat in the small intestine and adequate bile helps to neutralize the acidic semi-digested foods that arrive from the stomach into the small intestine. The flush helps to open the bile ducts, increases the flow of alkaline bile, which enhances digestion, and eliminates toxins from the liver.

Especially in the Leaky Gut Syndrome, the liver is very overworked trying to eliminate bacteria, parasites, toxins, and large food particles that leak through the small intestines (all which are acid-forming.) Persons with gallstones and a sluggish liver will probably have aches and pains over the liver area and shoulder blades and neck.

By doing a liver flush, it should dramatically improve digestion, help your energy level, help balance your pH, and eliminate the aches and pains. You might see many gallstones in the stool the next morning after the flush; they will be green or cream colored.

How to do the gallbladder/liver flush: [1]

- Choose a day like Saturday so you will be able to rest the next day.

- Eat a no-fat breakfast and lunch, this allows bile to build up and develop pressure. Higher pressure helps to increase the flow of bile and eliminate gallstones.

- Do not eat after 2 pm. You may drink water or apple juice.

- One hour before retiring drink one bottle of cold Magnesium Citrate, a laxative that can be purchased at a drug store. (It will taste better cold.)

- Right before laying down drink ¼ cup of olive oil (light olive oil tastes better) mixed with ½ cup of *fresh* pink grapefruit juice. It is best to mix the olive oil and juice in a jar with a lid, shake vigorously, and drink with a straw. Get it down within 5 minutes.

- Immediately lay down in bed on your left side with your head up high on a pillow. You might experience some nausea.

- Expect diarrhea in the morning, and expect to see gallstones in the stool.

- You may repeat the gallbladder/liver flush once a month until all the stones are eliminated.

[1] Adapted from Dr. Hulda Clark, Phd, ND, *The Cure for All Diseases*, San Diego: ProMotion Publishing, 1995, pp. 544-550

OSTEOPOROSIS

"It is bizarre that the produce manager is more important to my children's health than the pediatrician."

— Meryl Streep

Osteoporosis is most prevalent among postmenopausal women. The bones contain calcium and magnesium two of the body's major alkaline mineral reserves. When the body becomes overly acidic and the diet does not contain adequate calcium and magnesium, the calcium and other alkaline minerals are released from teeth and bones to keep the pH of the blood stable. Although, in the short run, this meets the blood's requirement to maintain the blood pH, bones become porous and brittle over time. This bone demineralization is one-reason persons as they age "shrink" in height. This is another reason it is so important to consume a high alkali-forming diet so that one consumes adequate calcium and magnesium to prevent bone demineralization and the factures that occur because of the loss of bone mass.

HORMONES

"Even one miracle cure can show the value of a therapy with the body's own healing powers. If the therapy is natural, non-invasive, and does no harm, it can be tried with confidence as a valid choice."

— Linda Rector-Page, ND, PhD

Briefly, menopause or "change of life" is the time when a woman stops ovulating or menstruating. When a woman stops ovulating, her ovaries decrease the production of the hormones estrogen and progesterone.

As stated earlier, hormones—or the lack thereof—affect the urinary system as well as the gynecological systems of a woman's body. Estrogen can drop by as much as 75% during menopause.

Estrogen helps stimulate the production of secretions that support the urinary system and the lubrication of the vagina. With the lack of estrogen one gets drying and thinning of the vagina and decreased secretions that protect the urinary system making the bladder more susceptible to infections.

Talking with an understanding gynecologist about hormone replacement therapy is an option that may increase the protective cellular layer inside the bladder and help with vaginal dryness. There are also different foods that are sources of natural plant estrogens. A good source book for natural supplements during menopause can be found in *Prescription for Nutritional Healing*, [1] by James Balch, MD, and Phyllis Balch, CNC.

[1] Phyllis A. Balch, CNC, and James Balch, MD, *Prescription for Nutritional Healing: A Practical A-Z Reference to Drug-Free Remedies Using Vitamins, Herbs, and Food Supplements,* 3rd and Revised Edition, New York: Avery Penguin Putnam, 2000

Sex

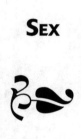

"The art of medicine consists in amusing the patient while nature cures the disease."

— Voltaire, French Philosopher (1694-1778)

I suggest for a week or two, when starting the alkali-forming diet, to choose alternative sexual outlets other than intercourse so that you can evaluate the diet with minimal painful interference. Once you are stable on the alkali-forming diet, explore different positions, and avoid the most painful ones at first. As your confidence builds with the diet, you can incorporate the positions that caused the most pain later.

Before starting my alkalizing program, I avoided the male-dominant missionary position because it caused more pain. I found the woman on top or penetration from behind or side-lying less painful. However, since I have changed to an alkalizing program, my symptom of cystitis after sex has disappeared. I am no longer worried about the usual painful aftermath I used to experience before I made these diet and lifestyle changes.

At various times, I used my allergy and inflammation homeopathics as well as MSM, bromelain, and papain after sex for flare-ups with excellent results. However, I cannot emphasize enough that maintaining an alkali-forming diet is what enabled me to resume normal sexual relations again without pain. The supplements are temporary measures. See Appendix F for more information regarding supplements.

In addition, we have enjoyed massages, creating intimate moments in the bath and shower, and finding a gentle and sensuous approach to intercourse more satisfying. Intimacy does not always have to mean sexual intercourse. Oral sex is not traumatic to the urinary tract and adds some surprise and diversity for those who are open to it.

Having adequate lubrication is important to decrease irritation to the uro-genital tract especially for peri- and post-menopausal women. A lubricant I like is called Slippery Stuff® Gel distributed by Wallace-O'Farrell. It contains no sugar that can contribute to yeast infections and looks and feels like one's natural lubrication. It is odorless and tasteless. Physician recommended Slippery Stuff® is a natural water-based lubrication that dissolves in water or natural body fluids thereby preventing bacterial or Candida growth. I apply a teaspoon or so into a vaginal applicator. I use the plastic applicator that came with a yeast medication for inserting vaginal suppositories and insert the gel into the vagina before intercourse. Remember to wash the applicator with soap and warm water in between applications and air dry.

Starting an Alkalizing Program

"Let thy medicine be thy food...and thy food thy medicine."

— Hippocrates

Although doctors are generally trained to use drugs, surgery, and the latest laboratory technologies, nutrition therapy is a real orphan in the medical community. In other words, to quote Abraham Maslow, "it is tempting, if the only tool you have is a hammer, to treat everything as if it were a nail." A true nutrition program has been overlooked in the treatment of IC. Diet changes and allergy elimination diets in the treatment of IC have been explored and with good results, but they have not gone far enough.

It is interesting to note, thus far, that doctors have reported an improvement of symptoms in those IC patients who observe certain food restrictions. The reported restrictions are acid-forming foods, allergens, and foods containing acids, such as chocolate and coffee, which contain tannic acid.

One could say with IC and, likely, other conditions that we have borrowed on our bodies' alkaline mineral stores, that we are essentially "bankrupt." With an alkali-forming diet/lifestyle we can restore, replenish, and eventually even start a "savings account" of alkalizing minerals.

Essentially, in my researching an alkalizing program, the studies recommend to consume 80% alkali-forming foods and 20% acid-forming foods. Foods that are alkalizing, fruits, vegetables, and dairy, contain calcium, potassium, iron, magnesium, and sodium. Foods that are acid-forming, meats and grains, contain phosphorus and sulfur.

Understand that eating a high acid diet is not the same thing as eating an acid-forming diet. Although they are high in citric acid, citrus fruits are metabolized, and they create an alkali ash in the body. In other words, fruits help to neutralize body acids. The potassium they contain is especially useful in neutralizing acids. However, persons with IC are troubled by the acid in foods, so there is a dilemma here. We need the alkaline elements found in fruit to help neutralize the body's acids, but we cannot tolerate the citric acid.

I discovered certain fruits less troublesome in the beginning of my alkalizing program. Pears, bananas, melons , papayas, and mangos have lower amounts of citric acid in them. In addition, once I was on my alkalizing program for a few months and my urine pH and saliva pH indicated my body trend was more alkaline with a pH between 7.0 and 7.4, I was able to consume citrus fruits and spicy foods with no "flare-ups." I was *not* taking any alkalizing supplements to tolerate these foods.

When making food choices, eat a variety of the freshest, organic seasonal fruits and vegetables as possible, preferably raw or lightly steamed from the neutral to highly alkalizing categories listed in the appendix. I wash and slice vegetables for a relish tray with ranch dressing or hummus that I serve with every evening meal along with a cooked vegetable or two and an entrée. Consider experimenting and adding new vegetables and fruits to your diet. Choose organic dairy and grain products without additives, hormones, and chemicals since these are toxins and acid-forming. Avoid sugar and salt since they are acidifying as well. Cooking fruits and vegetables decreases their alkalinity, and over-cooking causes them to be acidifying.

I have organized a list of foods and activities for the reader to explore. Briefly, I will present five essential alkali elements and the benefits they provide in the body, remembering there are other vitamins, minerals, essential fatty acids, and trace elements required, too. This is why it is so critical to eat a well-balanced alkali-forming diet.

"Every human being or animal that dies of 'natural causes' dies of a mineral deficiency."

— Nobel Prize nominee, Dr. Joel Wallach

Autonomic Nervous System

The sympathetic nervous system (SNS) in the body controls our fight or flight response mechanism. The parasympathetic system (PSNS) in the body controls our rest and digestive response mechanism. It works like this:

- Calcium: Stimulatory mineral for the Sympathetic Nervous System

- Magnesium: Inhibitory mineral for the Sympathetic Nervous System

- Potassium: Stimulatory mineral for the Parasympathetic Nervous System

- Sodium: Inhibitory mineral for the Parasympathetic Nervous System

Note that too much calcium and sodium are stimulating and that magnesium and potassium are relaxing to the body. Most Americans do not get sufficient calcium, but we are especially deficient in magnesium and potassium.

"Eight out of the top ten causes of death in the United States are the result of diet related degenerative diseases."

— Former US Surgeon General, Dr. C. Everett Koop, MD

Calcium
Stimulatory Mineral for the Sympathetic Nervous System

Calcium is one of the alkali elements needed to help neutralize and buffer our body's acids. Calcium is necessary with phosphorus to help build and maintain strong bones and teeth. About 99% of the body's calcium is found in the bones and teeth, and it is the most abundant mineral in the body. Adequate calcium is needed also for proper muscle contraction, nerve conduction, and blood clotting.

Proper absorption of calcium also depends on adequate amounts of vitamin D. Adequate amounts of the fat-soluble vitamin D can be ingested (400IU) or acquired by exposure to sunlight. 10 to 15 minutes of exposure to good sunlight without a sunscreen two to three times a week is sufficient.

Supplementation of up to 2500mg of calcium a day is considered safe. Calcium absorption is reported to be inefficient with only 20 to 30% absorbed. Your body can only absorb approximately 500mg of calcium at a time therefore it is recommended to take calcium in divided doses with meals and at bedtime for best absorption. If you take vitamin C that is buffered with calcium so it is not too acidic, make sure you count the milligrams of calcium in the buffered supplement so your calcium and magnesium intake are 1:1.

Too much phosphorus—found in carbonated beverages

and meat—also interferes with calcium absorption. It is recommended that phosphorus not exceed the amount of calcium taken.

In addition, calcium and magnesium compete for the same absorption sites. "In individuals with inflammatory conditions [like IC], the normal calcium to magnesium ratio of 2:1 can be modified to 1:1 or even 1:2." [1] Magnesium helps to relax muscles and helps to minimize allergic reactions. Calcium and magnesium are needed to properly maintain the heart and blood vessels.

Low levels of calcium intake are associated with increased risk of high blood pressure, fragile porous bones and osteoporosis, abnormal heartbeat, dementia, convulsions, nervous conditions, muscle cramps and numbness of the arms and legs.

When you have an inadequate intake of calcium the body will take the calcium from the bones starting with the spine and pelvis first; this is what thins the bones and causes osteoporosis and also causes us to "shrink" as we age. Dental problems and loss of teeth can be traced to inadequate calcium intake. Consuming more than three ounces of protein per day causes the body to excrete calcium.

Dairy foods are highest in calcium with the exception of cottage cheese. If you are dairy intolerant, there is calcium fortified orange juice or fortified soymilk. I enjoy chocolate soymilk. One cup of milk or yogurt or 1 ½ oz. of cheese provides about 300mg. of calcium. ½ cup of cooked broccoli, 1 oz. of almonds (about 30 almonds) or 1 tablespoon of molasses provides about 100mg. of calcium. Mineral supplements are also available.

The use of mineral supplements is recommended, since the average daily intake of calcium for most Americans is only about 400mg to 500mg per day. If the average intake of calcium is 500mg, and one consumes meat, coffee, sodas and alcohol that causes the excretion of alkaline elements in the urine, then most Americans have a negative balance of calcium. Calcium *carbonate* is an alkalizing calcium supplement. It should be taken in divided doses at mealtimes and before bed.

Calcium has a *stimulatory* effect on the sympathetic nervous system, responsible for fight or flight. In other words, calcium has a stimulating effect on the body.

The Daily Recommended Intake (DRI) of Calcium: [2]

- Age 51 and over: 1200mg because of reduced rate of absorption

- Adults ages 19 to 50: 1000mg;

- During pregnancy and lactation: 1000mg for women 19 and older; 1300mg for women 18 and younger;

- Preteens and teens ages 9 to 18: 1300mg;

- Children ages 4 to 8: 800mg;

- Children ages 1 to 3: 500mg;

- Infants ages 6 months to 1 year: 270mg;

- Newborn to age 6 months: 210mg

"You can trace every sickness, every disease, and every ailment to a mineral deficiency."

— Two-time Nobel Prize winner, Dr. Linus Pauling

Magnesium
Inhibitory mineral for the Sympathetic Nervous System

Nearly 70% of the body's supply of magnesium is located in the bones while 30% is found in the cellular fluids and some soft tissue.

Magnesium is involved in electrical stability of the cells, neurotransmission, and helps regulate the acid-alkali balance in the body. Evidence suggests that if calcium intake is high, magnesium intake needs to be high or there will be a deficiency of magnesium. *Magnesium helps promote absorption and metabolism of other minerals such as calcium, phosphorus, sodium, and potassium.*

It is estimated that the typical American diet barely meets the recommended daily amount of magnesium. Magnesium deficiency can easily occur because magnesium is refined out of many foods during processing. Cooking foods removes the minerals. A deficiency can occur in people with diabetes, persons on diuretics and digitalis medications, the elderly, those with pancreatitis, alcoholism, pregnancy, and those on low calorie diets and high carbohydrate diets.

Magnesium deficiency is thought to be closely related to coronary (heart) disease and strokes. Symptoms of a deficiency may include gastrointestinal disorders, irregular heart rhythm, lack of coordination, muscle twitch, tremors, weakness, apprehension, personality changes, confusion, depression, and irritability.

Potassium and magnesium (along with organic sodium) are some of the most important minerals for rebalancing the electrical properties of the cell and eliminating excess acidity and help to balance calcium.

Magnesium is found chiefly in fresh green vegetables and is an essential element in chlorophyll. I like to add *Veggie*

Magma™ (a powdered vegetable juice supplement) to tomato juice or apple juice for a great energy boost. Other excellent sources are soybeans, milk, whole grains, seafood, figs, corn, apples, and nuts, especially almonds.

Magnesium *inhibits* the sympathetic nervous system, responsible for fight or flight. In other words, magnesium has a calming effect on the body.

The Daily Recommended Intake (DRI) of Magnesium: [3]

- Adult males 31 to 70: 420mg;

- Adult females 31 to 70: 320mg;

- Adult males 19 to 30: 400mg;

- Adult females 19 to 30: 310mg;

- Pregnancy: add 40mg to comparable age;

- Lactation: same as comparable age;

- Males 14 to 18: 410mg;

- Females 14 to 18: 360mg;

- Children 9 to 13: 240mg;

- Children 4 to 8: 130mg;

- Toddlers 1 to 3: 80mg;

- Infants 6 months to 1: 75mg;

- Newborn to 6 months: 30mg

"I give you all the seed-bearing plants that are upon the earth, and all the trees with seed-bearing fruit; this shall be your food."

— Genesis 1:29

Potassium
Stimulatory Mineral for the Parasympathetic Nervous System

Potassium is an essential alkaline ion that is found mostly inside the cells (98%). Potassium and sodium together help regulate the distribution of body fluids. It unites with phosphorus to send oxygen to the brain, keeps skin healthy, stabilizes blood pressure, and works with sodium to keep the heartbeat regular. Potassium has been used to prevent and treat high blood pressure and has proved effective in treating allergies.

Potassium and magnesium (along with organic sodium) are some of the most important minerals for rebalancing the electrical properties of the cell and eliminating excess acidity and help to balance calcium.

Kidney failure or an inability to urinate causes toxicity. Hypokalemia or low potassium can also be caused by acute dehydration, adrenal insufficiency, and chronic renal failure. A low intake of potassium and a high intake of sodium can lead to hypertension.

The excessive use of table salt depletes the often-scarce potassium supplies. Diarrhea can deplete potassium levels and potassium stores decline with age. A potassium deficiency can result from an inadequate intake of fruits and vegetables. Mental and physical stress, diuretics, and diabetic acidosis can cause a large loss of potassium.

Some signs of potassium deficiencies are nervous disorders, insomnia, constipation, slow, irregular heartbeat, and impaired glucose metabolism.

In metabolic acidosis, H+ (hydrogen ions or acids) enter the inside of the cells while K+ (potassium ions) are "kicked" out of the cell and excreted in the urine. This is how the cells become acidic over time, and we deplete our alkaline buffer system, especially potassium. Bicarbonate raises the pH and reverses this H+ and K+ exchange process.

Good sources of potassium include all vegetables, especially green leafy ones, orange juice, bananas, avocadoes, potatoes (especially the skin), garlic, dried fruit, and apricots.

Potassium has a *stimulatory* effect on the calming parasympathetic nervous system. In other words, it has a relaxing effect on the body.

The Dietary Goals of the United States for potassium suggests: [4]

- § Adults and children 10 to 18: 2000mg;

- § Children 6 to 9: 1600mg;

- § Children 2 to 5: 1400mg;

- § Toddlers 1 to 2: 1000mg;

- § Infants 6 months to 1: 700mg;

- § Newborn to 6 months: 500mg

"Sowe Carrets in you Gardens, and humbly praise God for them, as for a singular and great blessing."

— Richard Gardiner, 1599

Sodium
Inhibitory mineral for the Parasympathetic Nervous System

Sodium is an essential mineral and is found in every cell in the body, but is predominately found in the extracellular fluids (fluids outside the cells).

Sodium functions with potassium to maintain the body's acid-alkaline balance. The usual intake in America far exceeds the need. An excess of sodium may lead to the loss of potassium and calcium in the body and may cause deficiencies. Diets that have an excess amount of sodium contribute to the rising incidences of liver, heart, and kidney disease.

Deficiencies are very uncommon because nearly all foods contain some sodium. The simplest way to reduce sodium intake is to eliminate the use of table salt. Plant sources have less sodium than animal sources, and processed foods are often very high in sodium.

Sodium *inhibits* the calming parasympathetic nervous system. In other words, sodium has a stimulating effect on the body.

The National Research Council recommends a daily sodium chloride intake for:

- Healthy adults: 1100mg to 3300mg;

- Children 10 to 18: 500 mg;

- Children 6 to 9: 400mg;

- Children 2 to 5: 300mg;

- Children 1 to 2: 225mg;

- Infants 6 months to 1: 200mg;

- Newborn to 6 months: 120mg;

"The whole is greater than the sum of its parts. Unlike supplements, fruits and vegetables contain a variety of nutrients, which cannot be extracted."

— Dr. T. Colin Campbell, PhD [5]

Iron

Iron is a mineral concentrate that is found in the largest amount in the blood. Iron is the main carrier vehicle for getting oxygen to all the cells of the body and helps in buffering acids in the body. Iron is needed to make hemoglobin, which carries oxygen from the lungs to all the tissues of the body.

Symptoms of deficiency as well as anemia may include constipation, lusterless or brittle nails, spoon-shaped nails, nail ridges that run lengthwise, difficulty breathing, tiredness, apathy, reduced brain function, pale pallor and heart enlargement.

Vitamin C increases the absorption of iron.

Some iron-rich foods are liver, oysters, and lean meat. Leafy green vegetables (especially spinach) whole grains, dried fruits, legumes, and molasses are rich in iron.

The Recommended Daily Allowance (RDA) of Iron: [6]

- Males 19 to 70: 10mg;

- Females 51 to 70: 10mg;

- Males 9 to 18: 12mg;

- Females 9 to 50: 15mg;

- Pregnancy: 30mg;

- Lactation: 15mg;

- Children 6 months to 8: 10mg;

- Newborn to 6 months: 6 mg

"The best interest of the patient is the only interest to be considered."

— Dr. William J. Mayo

Essential Fatty Acids

Essential fatty acids are fats that we need in our diets on a daily basis. We must consume these fats because our bodies do not manufacture them. There are two essential fats: linolenic acid (omega-3 family) and linoleic acid (omega-6 family.) These fats are necessary components of the membranes of all our cells in the body. They are required for proper brain development and function, vision and hearing.

"The brain is an astonishing 60 percent fat, and it needs omega-3s to function properly. In the last century, however, Americans have drastically reduced their intake of these oils, as we moved to diets based on processed foods. This deficit, scientists agree, has contributed to an epidemic of heart disease. Now a spate of cross-national studies has also linked low fish consumption to high rates of major depression, bipolar disorder, postpartum depression, and suicidal tendencies. 'Heart disease and depression often go hand in hand,' says Dr. Joseph Hibbeln, the National Institutes of Health psychiatrist who conducted a number of these surveys. 'Now we may know why.'

"While omega-3s are important for everyone, an adequate supply is especially critical for infants and mothers. Gestating and newborn babies often deplete their moms of these fats in order to nourish their own brains. If a woman is low on omega-3s to begin with, this depletion may set the stage for postpartum depression. A child takes in large amounts of these fats during the third trimester of gestation, and breast milk maintains a steady supply following birth. Infant formulas, by contrast, deliver very little.

"(The FDA, however, recently warned pregnant women against eating four types of fish with high mercury levels— shark, swordfish, tilefish and king mackerel.) Flaxseed, flaxseed oil, wheat germ and walnuts are good sources, too, as are dark greens such as spinach and kale. You can also boost your omega-3 levels by switching from corn and soybean oil to canola oil." [7]

Sources for linolenic acid (omega-3 family) are cold-water high fat fish such as salmon, trout, tuna, and mackerel. Fish oil capsules can be supplemented. Good plant sources are flaxseed oil, soybeans, pumpkin seeds, and walnuts.

Sources for linoleic acid (omega-6 family) are flaxseed oil, safflower oil, sunflower oil, and sesame seed oil.

I use a liquid supplement called *The Total EFA*™ (essential fatty acids) found in the refrigerated section of our health food store that I take daily with a chelated liquid vitamin and mineral supplement. I also make sure my family takes these vitamin-mineral and EFA supplements.

I know this may be off the subject of IC, but after six weeks of taking a daily liquid vitamin-mineral supplement and Total EFA™, my three-year-old son's tantrums and irritability are practically non-existent. He is far more cooperative and patient. I really notice a big change since we started the supplements. I mix it in chocolate milk because he enjoys that. Since it is a known fact children don't always choose to eat the most nutritious food one could mix the supplements in drinks, yogurt, smoothies, and pudding over the course of the day and evening to ensure adequate essential nutrients.

Daily Values for Everyone

The 1990 Nutrition Labeling and Education Act brought us Daily Values on food labels beginning in 1994. Before this time, our food labels listed percentages of the US RDA. Actually, the Daily Values combine the old US RDA, renamed Reference Daily Intake, and a set of standards called Daily Reference Value (DRV) for other nutrients. The only term that appears on the label, however, is Daily Value. This information is presented below.

Daily Values = Daily Reference Values + Reference Daily Intakes

Table 4: Reference Daily Intakes

Reference Daily Intakes	Adults & Children Aged 4 or Older
Vitamin A, IU	5000
Vitamin C, mg	60
Calcium, g	1
Iron, mg	18
Vitamin D, IU	400
Vitamin E, IU	30
Vitamin K, mcg	80
Thiamin, mg	1.5
Riboflavin, mg	1.7
Niacin, mg	20
Vitamin B6, mg	2
Folic Acid, mg	0.4

Table 4: Reference Daily Intakes (con't)

Reference Daily Intakes	Adults & Children Aged 4 or Older
Vitamin B12, mcg	6
Biotin, mg	0.3
Pantothenic acid, mg	10
Phosphorus, g	1
Iodine, mcg	150
Magnesium, mg	400
Zinc, mg	15
Selenium, mcg	70
Copper, mg	2
Manganese, mg	2
Chromium, mcg	120
Molybdenum, mcg	75

Table 5: Daily Reference Values

Daily Reference Values	Based on 2,000 calorie intake
Total Fat, g	65
Saturated Fat, g	20
Cholesterol, mg	300
Total Carbohydrate, g	300
Dietary Fiber, g	25
Sodium, mg	2400
Potassium, mg	3500
Protein, g	50

Dietary Guidelines

"On February 23, 1999 a coalition of more than 20 groups, including the American Heart Association, The American Cancer Society, The Produce for Better Health Foundation (PBH), the American Institute for Cancer Research, the Boys & Girls Clubs of America, the American Diabetes Association and the American Association of Retired Persons urged the government to make fruits and vegetables the center of the American diet. This message was primarily directed to the members of the Dietary Guidelines Committee, who are making up the nutritional guidelines to be revised for the year 2000.

"The groups say there is strong evidence that if people eat more fruits and vegetables, lives and a considerable amount of health care dollars will be saved. According to this group, five of the top ten causes of death in the United States are diet related—heart disease, cancer, strokes, diabetes, and other forms of atherosclerosis, and diet plays a preventive role in birth defects, cataract formation, hypertension, asthma, diverticulosis, obesity, and diabetes.

"Talking about Americans... 'Dinnertime is vegetable time; over 75% of all vegetables they eat are consumed at this time. But, even though dinnertime is the most popular time for eating fruits and vegetables, only 28% of the foods they eat at dinner are fruits, vegetable, or 100% juices. The average American's annual fruit and vegetable deficit is serious,' ... 'Most of us have an annual fruit and vegetable deficit ranging from 219 to 1,629 servings—that's per person. It really adds up.'" [8]

The position of the American Dietetic Association is that appropriately planned vegetarian diets are healthful, are nutritionally adequate, and provide health benefits in the prevention and treatment of certain diseases. According to the

ADA, mortality rates are lower in vegetarians for the following diseases: coronary artery disease, hypertension, lung and colorectal cancer, and cross-cultural data indicates lower breast cancer rates. The Vegetarian Diet Pyramid can be used for a healthy standard to follow for an alkalizing program.

I am not suggesting the reader needs to become a vegetarian; I am merely presenting the information available on known diets as they relate to disease prevention.

Researchers from Harvard, Oldways, and the World Health Organization have developed the Traditional Healthy Mediterranean Diet Pyramid. This pyramid reflects the current state of worldwide clinical and epidemiological research on healthy eating and low rates of diet-linked chronic diseases and high life expectancy typical of the Mediterranean region in 1960. The Mediterranean diet pyramid may be used as a guide for those of you who wish more structure in an alkalizing program.

This diet is a good example of an alkalizing diet high in the alkalizing elements such as iron, calcium, potassium, magnesium and breaks down to the basics:

- Eat low to moderate amounts of cheese and yogurt.

- Eat minimally processed, seasonally fresh, and locally grown foods.

- Consume an abundance of foods from plant sources including fruits and vegetables, potatoes, beans, nuts and seeds, grains.

- Consume low to moderate amounts of fish and poultry weekly; limit eggs to zero to four servings per week.

- Eat fruit as a typical daily dessert.

- Only eat red meat a few times per month.

§ Use olive oil as the principal fat replacing other fats and oils.

§ Total dietary fat should range from 25% to 35% of energy, with saturated fat no more than 7 to 8 percent of total calories.

§ Drink only a moderate amount of wine normally with meals—about one to two glasses per day for men and one glass per day for women. [9]

§ Incorporate regular physical activity at a level that promotes healthy weight, fitness, and well-being.

When making food selections try to choose a variety of different fruits, vegetables, legumes, nuts, seeds, and grains. This will increase the essential trace elements needed. Select as close to eighty percent of your food from the neutral to high alkali-forming categories listed in the appendix of this book, with emphasis at every meal on fruits and vegetables. When choosing fish, consider the high omega-3 sources such as salmon, tuna, mackerel, trout, halibut, whitefish, sardines, anchovy, orange roughie, or bluefish. Eat shellfish rarely since they live in the most polluted waters close to shore.

If you enjoy eating meat, choose free-ranging organic poultry or meat that has not been subjected to hormones or antibiotics. However, studies show that the amount of protein eaten can lower your calcium levels. Protein intake of over three ounces a day causes a loss of calcium from the urinary tract.

It is important to eat a well-balanced diet to consume adequate daily trace elements, vitamins, minerals, fiber, and essential fatty acids. One goal of an alkali-forming diet plan is to replace the lost minerals. Youths are naturally quite alkaline, which is why one sees so much exuberance and energy. Theoretically, I suppose you could regain the vitality of youth

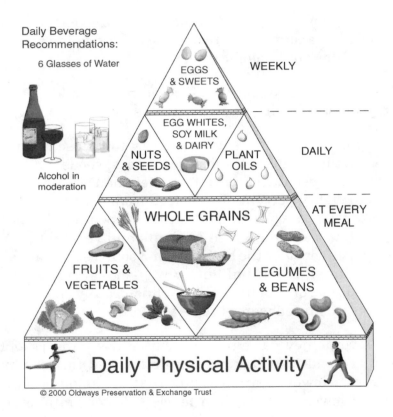

The Traditional Healthy
Vegetarian Diet Pyramid

Daily Beverage Recommendations:

6 Glasses of Water

Alcohol in moderation

WEEKLY

EGGS & SWEETS

EGG WHITES, SOY MILK & DAIRY

NUTS & SEEDS

PLANT OILS

DAILY

WHOLE GRAINS

AT EVERY MEAL

FRUITS & VEGETABLES

LEGUMES & BEANS

Daily Physical Activity

by following an alkalizing program. It is important with children to maintain their alkaline stores by encouraging plenty of fruits, vegetables, and calcium daily. It is essential to avoid caffeine and sodas and limit sugary or salty snacks. Refer to Table 6 on page 151 for some suggested food substitutions for

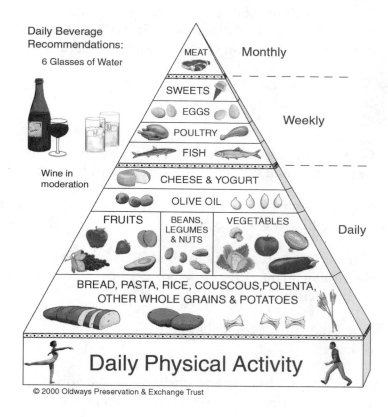

The Traditional Healthy Mediterranean Diet Pyramid

Daily Beverage Recommendations:

6 Glasses of Water

Wine in moderation

MEAT — Monthly

SWEETS

EGGS

POULTRY — Weekly

FISH

CHEESE & YOGURT

OLIVE OIL

FRUITS | BEANS, LEGUMES & NUTS | VEGETABLES — Daily

BREAD, PASTA, RICE, COUSCOUS, POLENTA, OTHER WHOLE GRAINS & POTATOES

Daily Physical Activity

© 2000 Oldways Preservation & Exchange Trust

children and adults to help make a more comfortable transition to an alkali-forming diet.

Foods to Avoid or Limit

The following acid-forming items are consumed in substantial quantities in the typical American diet. These items are troublesome to persons with IC and increase "flare-ups."

Cola drinks (pH 2.5) (addictive, mood and energy altering)

- Caffeine (50mg per serving) creates a diuretic effect causing the kidneys to excrete the alkalizing elements calcium, magnesium, sodium, and potassium.

- The diuretic effect of caffeine increases urination and the drying of the mucosa in the vagina, urethra, and bladder.

- Caffeine stimulates the production of hydrochloric acid in the stomach, which adds to the acid load of the body.

- Sugar with caffeine doubles the amount of calcium excreted by the kidneys.

- Carbonation in soda is formed by adding carbon dioxide. Carbon dioxide is an acid that adds to the body's acid load.

- The kola nut of the cola acuminata has a stimulatory effect that intensifies physiological responses to stress.

Coffee (pH 5) (addictive, mood and energy altering)

- Coffee contains over 208 kinds of acids.

- Caffeine (100mg per cup) causes a diuretic effect that causes the kidneys to excrete the alkalizing elements calcium, magnesium, sodium, and potassium.

- The diuretic effect of caffeine increases urination and the drying of mucosa in the vagina, urethra, and bladder.

- Caffeine stimulates the increase production of hydrochloric acid in the stomach, which adds to the acid load in the body.

- Sugar in a cup of coffee doubles the amount of calcium excreted by the kidneys.

- Caffeine intensifies physiological responses to stress.

Black Tea pH (pH 6.5) (addictive, mood and energy altering)

- Caffeine 60 mg per cup causes a diuretic effect that causes the kidneys to excrete the alkalizing elements, including calcium, magnesium, sodium, and potassium.

- The diuretic effect of caffeine increases urination and the drying of mucosa in the vagina, urethra, and bladder.

- Caffeine stimulates the increase production of hydrochloric acid in the stomach, which adds to the acid load in the body.

- Caffeine intensifies physiological responses to stress.

Alcohol (addictive, mood and energy altering)

- Alcohol has poor nutritive value except calories.

- The diuretic effect causes the kidneys to excrete the alkalizing elements, including calcium and magnesium.

- The diuretic effect also causes drying of the mucosa of the vagina, urethra, and bladder.

Sugar (addictive, mood and energy altering)
§ Sugar depletes the body of B-complex vitamins and
alkaline minerals increasing anxiety and irritability.

Carbonated Beverages
§ All carbonated or sparkling drinks contain carbon
dioxide an acid.

Salt
§ Excess salt causes the excretion of potassium.

Stress and the Adrenal Glands
*"Any stressor that the mind or body interprets and internalizes
as too much to deal with, leaves an acid residue. Even a mild
stressor can cause a partial or total acid-forming reaction."*

— Dr. Theodore A. Baroody

Most Americans spend more time producing acid waste
products especially related to stress than processing it. Stress
is acid-forming. The two adrenal glands situated on top of each
kidney produce hormones in response to stress. These hormones
are responsible for the fight or flight response in the body.

Table 6: Food Substitutions

Acidifying Food	More Alkalizing Substitute
Wheat Crackers or Bread	Rice, Soy, Rye, Corn, Oat, Spelt, Millet
Chocolate Chip Cookie	Fig or Raisin Cookie
Peanut Butter Crackers	Nut Butter on Rice Cracker
Salted Nuts	Dry Roasted Almonds, Nuts, or Seeds
Salted Chips	Salt-Free/Low Salt Chips or Vegetable Sticks
Sour Cream Dip	Hummus, Guacamole, Salsa
Milk Shake	Fruit Smoothie
Ice Cream	Yogurt Topped with Fruit, Rice /Soy Frozen Desserts
Spaghetti Meat Sauce	Soy-based Italian Meatless Sauce
Wheat Pasta	Vegetable Pastas, Rice or Lentil Pastas
Sausage Pizza	Spinach or Vegetable Pizza
Beef Stew	Minestrone Soup
Burger Fast Food	Vegetable Chow Mein, Vegetable Burrito
Coffee	Coffee Substitutes, Ginger Tea
Carbonated Water	Alkaline Water
Soda	Fruit Juice, Alkaline Water
Pretzels	Reduced Salt Popcorn
Candy	Dried Fruit
French Fries	Sweet or Baked Potato
Sugar	Honey, Molasses, Maple Syrup
Salt	Low Salt or Salt Substitute, Sea Vegetables, or Herbs
Black or Green Tea	Herbal Teas, Especially Ginger Tea

In a stressful situation, these adrenal hormones:

- Transfer blood from the intestines to the extremities;

- Increase blood pressure;

- Increase your heart rate;

- Suppress the immune system;

- Increase the blood's clotting ability

There are different types of stress:

- Emotional
- Thermal
- Physical
- Chemical

Emotional stress can be positive or negative. For example, a promotion at work might be a positive one and an IRS audit a negative one. In either case, the excitement elicited from these changes still affects the adrenal glands. *Thermal stress* comes from being exposed to extreme temperatures. *Physical stress* can be from heavy physical work, lack of sleep, living a sedentary life style, or being overweight. *Chemical stress* can be from exposure to caffeine, pollutants, and rapid changes in blood sugar levels from sugar consumption.

Sustained stress from worry, caffeine, sugar, etc. can decrease the immune system causing a person to be sick often or develop allergies. Continued stress can cause decreased blood flow to the bowels and create digestive problems such as LGS or irritable bowel.

Adrenal hormones cause an increase in blood clotting which can lead to arterial plaquing and heart disease. The adrenal glands do not know the difference between the stress produced by a cup of coffee or from being laid off at work.

Eventually, accumulated stress wears out the adrenal glands, they fail to meet the demands, and varieties of symptoms include fatigue, digestive problems, obesity, depression, allergies, and over acidity of the body.

People with weak adrenal glands crave caffeine and sugar because these substances stimulate the adrenal glands that are failing. What you need is rest, relaxation, and proper nourishment. Eliminating stress wherever possible will go a long way to helping heal the adrenal glands and alkalize the body.

Although an alkali-forming diet is very important as a base in an alkalizing program it is important to address stress factors in one's life. Being more aware of stress and exploring ways to eliminate or cope better with stress is a good starting point. Please consider the list of alkali-forming versus acid-forming lifestyle choices in the appendix as a starting point for some life changes.

Pantothenic Acid

The body relies on Pantothenic acid to help the adrenal glands produce stress hormones during times of both psychological and physical strain. This property makes it potentially useful for dealing with emotional upset, depression, anxiety, migraines, chronic fatigue, and withdrawal from alcohol or tobacco. It is commonly taken as part of a vitamin B complex supplement for these purposes.

Allergy sufferers may find Pantothenic acid beneficial for controlling the nasal congestion that can develop during an allergic reaction. An asthmatic response initiated by seasonal allergies may similarly improve with Pantothenic acid. There is no formal RDA for Pantothenic acid. There are no known drug or nutrient interactions associated with Pantothenic acid.

For psychological or physical stress: Take a daily vitamin B complex supplement that includes 100 mg of Pantothenic acid. Many so-called adrenal support combinations designed to help the body cope with stress contain approximately this amount of Pantothenic acid. Take Pantothenic acid with meals.

Suggested Dosages of Pantothenic Acid
- For Stress, take 100mg per day.

- For allergies, take 500mg of Pantothenic acid three times a day.

- For Chronic Fatigue Syndrome, take 500mg twice a day.

Yeast Infections (Candida albicans)
If you currently have a systemic yeast infection, I encourage you to read *The Yeast Connection* by Dr. William G. Crook, MD. It is an excellent resource to help you overcome your yeast infection. I would caution you to eat only your daily protein requirements. The yeast connection diet consists of a majority of vegetables, so if you are careful with your protein intake, you can resolve your yeast problem as well as alkalizing yourself.

Protein
Protein is needed to build and repair body tissues. The recommended protein intake for adults, on average, is 0.8 grams of protein per kilogram (kg) of body weight. If you add intense weight training, this amount can climb to 1.2 - 1.6 grams per kg body weight. However, the regular consumption of protein in the U.S. exceeds the recommended daily amount for regular or body building needs, so most people don't need to add more protein-rich foods to their daily intake.

If you choose a vegetarian diet, you need to know that plants have different amino acid (the building blocks of protein) patterns and offer less protein per unit than animal foods. Animal proteins provide complete amino acids... the ones we need to build our protein. Plants supply incomplete proteins, but by eating various plant groups, a person can get the amino acids they need. These do not have to be eaten at the same time, or in the same meal, but they need to be eaten sometime during the same day. Examples of plant protein combinations to get complete amino acids include beans and rice; peanut butter and bread; and, tofu, stir-fried vegetables, and rice. Soy protein is complete by itself. As a general rule, legumes with grains or nuts with grains provide you with complete amino acids. So will eggs and milk products.

Supplements

The following supplements have been shown to greatly reduce IC symptoms. [10]

For Interstitial Cystitis

Sodium bicarbonate is a nontoxic white powder that is used commonly as a leavening agent, cleanser, and antacid. The pH of sodium bicarbonate or baking soda is 8.3. Suggested dosage for IC symptoms: ¼ to ½ teaspoon mixed in 4 oz water every hour or two until symptoms subside. Sodium bicarbonate can be purchased at a grocery store.

Potassium bicarbonate is a white non-toxic powder and can be used in an alkalizing program. Potassium bicarbonate is found in nutritional supplements. It is recommended to take in combination with sodium bicarbonate. It is preferable to take sodium bicarbonate and potassium bicarbonate in combination in a ratio of 4:1 or 8:1. (Four parts sodium bicarbonate to one part potassium bicarbonate or eight parts sodium bicarbonate to one part potassium bicarbonate.) A pharmacist can mix this combination or individuals can mix a small amount for themselves. I mixed a 4:1 ratio and used it occasionally in the beginning of my alkalizing program. Potassium bicarbonate can only be purchased at a chemical supply house. Buy USP grade. (US Pharmacopoeia grade)

Sodium bicarbonate and potassium bicarbonate should be taken in a 4:1 or 8:1 ratio. For inflammatory conditions suggested dosage: ¼ to ½ teaspoon mixed with 4 oz water three to four times per day thirty minutes before a meal or two hours after a meal.

Sodium citrate helps to alkalize the urine, but does not alkalize the entire body. Sodium citrate has been used to relieve bacterial and interstitial cystitis and to relieve indigestion. Sodium citrate can be use in combination with sodium bicarbonate in relieving IC symptoms. Sodium bicarbonate can be taken for more immediate relief of IC. Sodium citrate is slower acting than sodium bicarbonate. Sodium citrate can be used for sustained relief from IC symptoms. Suggested dosage for IC is ½ to ¾ teaspoon in 4 oz of water twice a day. Sodium citrate can be ordered from health food stores. Buy USP grade (US Pharmacopoeia grade).

Warnings and Precautions

You may not be able to take potassium bicarbonate, sodium bicarbonate or sodium citrate if you have kidney or heart disease or high blood pressure; are taking a potassium sparing diuretic; have Addison's disease; have a stomach ulcer or intestinal blockage; or have chronic diarrhea. If you are pregnant or nursing a baby, do not take any supplements without consulting your health care provider. Medications can compound the effects of the supplements and certain medical conditions may contraindicate the use of any supplements so consult your health care provider before starting supplements.

Taking too much sodium or potassium bicarbonate can make you too alkaline. Some signs and symptoms of being too alkaline are these: feeling overly energized, unable to sleep, tingling in the arms, hands, legs, and lips as well as feeling anxious.

Severe overdosing can result in muscle spasms or tetany, which can start in the forearms and spread throughout the body. Muscle spasms in the chest that effect breathing can be **fatal**. Bicarbonate can cause bloating or gas in some individuals.

If you experience any of these symptoms, reduce the dosage and frequency of sodium and potassium bicarbonate.

To reduce alkalosis, drinking coffee, black tea, lemonade, or cola drinks will cause the body to become more acidic and restore your pH balance. Vigorous exercise also will increase acidity.

It is important to take sodium and potassium bicarbonate 30 minutes before a meal or two hours after a meal so the supplement does not interfere with digestion since it will neutralize stomach acids temporarily which is not good for the digestion.

When taking sodium and potassium bicarbonate or sodium citrate start with the lowest dose recommended to obtain symptom relief. Remember that the supplements are only for symptom relief and an alkali-forming diet and lifestyle changes are needed to make long-term corrections of acid-alkali imbalances. I personally only used sodium and potassium bicarbonate 4:1 supplement one dose every other week for the first couple months. I strongly encourage maintaining an alkali-forming diet over supplements, as it is healthier and safer.

For Inflammatory Conditions

MSM (methylsulfonylmethane) is a powerful anti-inflammatory derived from natural foods. It is an FDA-approved treatment for interstitial cystitis. It is also *anti-parasitic* and *antifungal*, which is believed to block the binding sites for parasites in the intestines (which helps with LGS) and uro-genital tract. The suggested dosage is 250mg to 750mg of MSM taken three times per day in divided doses with meals. MSM can be purchased at health food stores.

Bromelain is derived from a natural plant source in the stem of the pineapple. Bromelain is an enzyme that acts as a natural aspirin without any side effects. It reduces inflammation. For inflammation, suggested dosage is 500mg taken two to four times per day apart from meals for inflammation. It should not be taken by pregnant women or persons with bleeding disorders. Bromelain can be purchased at health food stores.

Papain is derived form papayas. It is an enzyme, and along with Bromelain is a useful treatment of inflammatory conditions. For inflammation, suggested dosage is 200mg to 300mg with or immediately following meals, upon rising, and before bedtime. It should not be taken by pregnant women or persons with bleeding disorders. Papain can be purchased at health food stores.

Example of an alkali-forming day —80% Alkali and 20% Acid:

- § Take Clear® anti-parasitic/anti-yeast supplement on empty stomach with a glass of alkaline water

- § Thirty minutes after taking Clear® take probiotics.

- Exercise: Start day with deep breathing and a yoga set or a morning walk

- Breakfast: Drink a fruit smoothie with sprouted grain muffin; take vitamins, minerals and essential fatty acid supplements

- Morning Snack: Vegetable juice with rye crackers and cheese

- Lunch: Vegetable soup with corn muffin and take a brisk 15-minute walk

- Afternoon Snack: Vegetable or fruit juice with *Veggie Magma*™ supplement for an energy boost and a handful of almonds

- Dinner: Salmon with baked potato and steamed green beans, fresh vegetable relish tray, and fruit for dessert

- Exercise: Evening stroll after dinner

- Evening Snack: Yogurt before bed

- Relaxation, massage, reading, bath, or meditation before sleep

- Drink 6 to 8 glasses of alkaline water.

Example of an acid-forming day —80% Acid and 20% Alkali:

- Breakfast: Two or three cups of coffee with cream and sugar, juice and a croissant or bagel

- Morning Snack: carbonated beverage with chips

- Lunch: rushed, with a fast food cheeseburger, french fries, and another carbonated beverage

- Afternoon Snack: coffee and chocolate chip cookies for an "energy boost"

- Exercise: running several miles or no exercise

- Alcoholic drink before dinner

- Dinner: Wine, steak with rice and peas, bread and butter, dinner salad

- Evening Snack: Chocolate brownie for dessert

- Stay up late to work or watch TV

- Drinks sodas and carbonated water throughout the day

[1] Lark, *Op. Cit.*, p. 248.

[2] These data are current as of 1998.

[3] These data are current as of 1998.

[4] No Daily Recommended Intake (DRI) for Potassium has been published.

[5] Dr. Campbell of Cornell University speaking for the American Institute for Cancer Research

[6] These data are current as of 1989.

[7] http://www.msnbc.com/news/559436.asp

[8] Dr. John McDougall, MD, http://www.drmcdougall.com/debate.html

[9] Persons with IC generally do not tolerate wine. Wine is acid-forming because of its diuretic effect, which causes urinary excretion of the alkalizing elements, including calcium and magnesium.

ALKALINE WATER

"The cell is immortal. It is merely the fluid in which it floats that degenerates. Renew this fluid at intervals, give the cells what they require for nutrition, and as far as we know, the pulsation of life may go on for ever."

— Dr. Alexis Carrel

What Is Pure Water?

We know that all life is dependent on water and that water exists in nature in many forms: clouds, rain, snow, ice, and fog; however, strictly speaking, chemically pure water does not exist for any appreciable length of time in nature. Even while falling as rain, water picks up small amounts of gases, ions, dust, and particulate matter from the atmosphere. Then, as it flows over or through the surface layers of the earth, it dissolves and carries with it some of almost everything it touches, including that which is dumped into it by man.

These substances include industrial and commercial solvents, pesticides, herbicides, radioactive materials, road salts, decaying animal and vegetable matter, and living microorganisms, such as algae, bacteria, and virus. These impurities may damage growing plants and transmit disease. Many of these impurities are removed or rendered harmless, however, in municipal drinking water treatment plants. Chlorine is the most widely used disinfectant for treating the water supply in the nation, with over half a million tons used annually by the water treatment industry. However, chlorine is an acid-forming element that has long-term negative health risks. It makes sense to filter tap water eliminating this acid-forming element and convert it to health-enhancing pure alkaline water with a pH as high as 9 to 11.

Table 7: The World's Water Supply [1]

Percentage of Total Global Reserve		
	Percentage of All Water	**Percentage of Fresh Water**
World Oceans	96.5	0
Glaciers and Permanent Snow	1.7	68.7
Groundwater	1.7	30.1
Ground Ice and Permafrost	0.02	0.9
Lakes	0.01	0.3
Soil Moisture	0.001	0.1
Atmosphere	0.001	0.04
Swamps	0.001	0.03
Rivers	0.0002	0.01
Plants	0.0001	0.003
Total	**100%**	**100%**

Ionized Alkaline Microwater

When water comes out of your tap, it tends to be grouped in clusters of approximately ten to thirteen water molecules. When water is bouncing off the rocks in a high mountain stream, picking up electrons, it tends to group together in smaller clusters of five to six water molecules making it smaller water or "micro-clustered" water. Hence, you have water that is one half the size, or "wetter" water. The negatively charged electrode in a micro-water machine draws to itself the alkaline minerals: sodium, potassium, calcium, and magnesium, creating water similar to that found in areas that are home to the healthiest and longest-lived people. The positively charged electrode attracts the acidic materials, the chlorides, sulfur compounds, and the H+ ions.

Ionized water is fundamentally different from conventional water. This is because the water molecule cluster has been reduced in size and the shape has been changed to hexagonal, the combination of which allows the water cluster to pass through our tissues more easily.

Water is one of the most important elements in the body, which is comprised of approximately seventy percent water. One of the contributing factors of chronic disease is not providing the body with sufficient alkaline water. Most individuals do not drink alkaline water nor are we properly hydrated. To calculate adequate fluid intake, take your weight, in pounds, divide it by two, and you will have approximately the number of fluid ounces you require daily:

Daily Intake of Water: 140lb $\div$ 2 = 70 fl. oz.

Alkaline Water Ionizer

In household sink ionizers, the water is first filtered through an activated carbon filter that removes chlorine, bacteria, and other pollutants but retaining the dissolved minerals. The water is then subjected to an electrical charge using electrolysis, which charges the water with positive and negative ions. The positive ions are the acidic minerals, which are bled off to one side leaving the beneficial alkaline minerals. These are the negative ion minerals such as calcium, magnesium, and potassium. These negative ions are extremely beneficial in neutralizing free radicals. Increased alkalinity is beneficial in neutralizing acidity in the body and transporting calcium to the bones. The ionizer does not add any chemicals or minerals to the water. It only splits the minerals already in the water to the alkali side and the acid side.

The objective of water ionizers is simple. The concept is to convert ordinary tap water into water similar to the natural tumbling waters of mountain streams and waterfalls. This water has a negative charge, which increases alkalinity. You might have noticed how beautiful the air is after a thunderstorm, and how invigorating the air is to breathe. This is because the air has been charged with negative ions. In much the same way, negative ions in the alkaline water you drink are also invigorating.

In Asia, they have been making water ionizers for more than thirty years with full approval of the Japanese and Korean ministries of health. Ionizers have been tested and approved by independent laboratories to meet FDA standards and are now sold in the US and UK markets.

The makers of the water unit state the cost of a water ionizing system is between $500 and $800 to purchase and should last approximately 10 years. [2] The maker's claim no plumber is required, it is simple to install, and the approximate cost of making pure, filtered, ionized water is about 2 cents per gallon. There are companies that produce units that treat the entire home water supply as well.

Oxygen

According to *Alternative Medicine Digest, Issue #9*, Dr. Hidemistu Hayashi, MD, is one of Japan's foremost Microwater (alkaline water) researchers. Dr. Hayashi says that alkaline Microwater acts as a powerful antioxidant in the body destroying harmful free radicals. In addition, once the body's cells absorb Microwater, says Dr. Hayashi, it helps dissolve acidic wastes that have accumulated over many years.

An antioxidant quality of ionized alkaline water is hydroxyl ions. These are oxygen molecules with an extra electron attached to them as are all antioxidants such as vitamins A, C, and E. Hydroxyl ions scavenge for free radicals, which are unstable oxygen molecules that cause damage to us. Once the hydroxyl antioxidant and free radical have canceled each other, the result is that the body is provided with lots of oxygen and therefore lots of energy.

Oxygen is the most abundant element on earth. Oxygen constitutes about two thirds of the human body and nine tenths (by weight) of the water in rivers, lakes, and oceans. Oxygen destroys cancer cells as well as bacteria and virus invading the body. Oxygen is one of the most exhausted nutrients in our body because of our diet and the earth's oxygen-depleted environment today. Since oxygen is an alkaline element, it helps to neutralize our body's acids. It is vital to human health, perhaps our most important nutrient.

How is Alkaline Water Different?

Alkaline water is different from the water we drink. It is called "living water" and contains negative ions, it has a different boiling point, freezing point, viscosity, surface tension, and can enter the cells three times faster.

Alkaline water has excess oxygen, more than the two to one ratio of ordinary water. The ionizer does not grab oxygen molecules from the air and put them in the alkaline water. What happens is that as the positively charged alkaline minerals come across the membrane into the alkaline chamber, they kick out one hydrogen atom from a water molecule, and it joins with hydroxyl ions (OH-). The hydrogen ions (H+) that have been kicked out receive an electron from the negative electrode to be de-ionized and become a hydrogen molecule (H_2) and bubble out of the water. In the acid chamber, the reverse phenomena take place. The millivoltage of alkaline water is lower. This means that the water molecule is re-figured into a lighter, simpler form. Restructured alkaline water alkalizes by displacing acid and replacing alkali.

Potential Benefits of the Alkaline Water Component of Ionization

- Increases energy level—related to increased alkali electrolytes and oxygen

- Washes acidic waste from the body

- Helps digestion, digestive problems, and promotes regularity

- Hydrates your body three times more effectively than conventional water or bottled water

- Nutrients are absorbed more efficiently into the body

- Food cooked with ionized water tastes better

- Makes food taste sweeter without adding sugar

- Powders such as flour are mixed more thoroughly and smoothly

- Ionized water boils faster and cools down faster

- Drinking alkaline water promotes healthier skin and complexion

- Good for animals as well as humans

- Healthy cells live in an alkalized environment

- Promotes overall health and healing by bringing the body into balance

Potential Benefits of Acid Water Component of Ionization—Do Not Drink

- Washing with acid water is good for complexion (Skin pH is 4.5 to 6)

- Wash food with it to remove bacteria

- Beneficial as a vaginal douche for Candida

- Helps to heal cuts, blisters, scrapes, or rashes

- Disinfects cutting boards, counters and utensils

- Treats fungi such as athlete's foot

- Provides excellent relief from mosquito bites, bee stings, poison ivy, or poison oak

- Makes a good hair rinse

- Effectively removes plaque from teeth, use it instead of toothpaste, *but rinse with alkaline water afterwards*

- Gargle with it to relieve sore throats or other mouth sores

- Works as an astringent for the skin

- Helps in the treatment of acne and eczema

- Promotes plant growth and their general health

- Extends the life of cut flowers

If the cost of a water ionizer is prohibitive, one can purchase a patented alkaline concentrate—a correct ratio of potassium and sodium—to provide alkalinity. One alkaline concentrate to consider is Alkalife® a water additive developed by scientist, engineer, and inventor Sang Whang, author of *Reverse Aging*.[3] He claims by simply adding two drops to an 8 to 10 oz glass of drinking water it will change ordinary drinking water into healthy alkaline water.

[1] Adapted from Igor A. Shildomanov, in *Water in Crises: A Guide to the World's Fresh Water Resources*, P. Gleick, ed., Oxford Univ. Press, N.Y., 1993

[2] Refer to the appendix for details.

[3] Sang Whang, *Reverse Aging*, Miami: JSP Publishing, 2000

CONCLUSION

"That which is above is the same as that which is below."

— Hermes Trismegistus

In solving the IC puzzle, I was reminded that the body is a microcosm of our natural external environment. It is important to view ones health holistically. By this, I mean exploring and altering ones diet is vital in resolving IC. As such, while my emphasis has been on maintaining an alkaliforming diet/lifestyle, it is important to remember that we all exist within a macrocosm. While researching information for my recovery from IC, I discovered the parallels of the acidification of our bodies and that of our world. We eat acid-forming food, drink water, and breathe air that has been exposed to acid deposition. To understand IC and acidity more thoroughly, we need to explore the world in which we live.

Parallels

While searching for information about "acid water" on the Internet, I came across myriad websites regarding the effects of acid rain. I was saddened by the devastating acidic conditions of the world's fresh-water lakes, rivers, streams, and wetlands. The devastation is particularly prevalent in Norway, Sweden, and Canada. However, the lakes and rivers of the United States have not been spared. "In the United States acid-sensitive areas are found in Minnesota, Wisconsin, upper Michigan, several Southeastern states, the mountainous areas of the West, as well as the Northeastern states.

"Other acid-sensitive parts of the world include the Netherlands, Belgium, Denmark, Switzerland, Italy, West Germany, Ireland, the United Kingdom, Scandinavia, and in the Precambrian and Cambrian geology in Asia, Africa, and South America."[1]

Acid Rain

"When fossil fuels such as coal, gasoline, and fuel oils are burned, they emit oxides of sulfur, carbon, and nitrogen into the air. These oxides combine with moisture in the air to form sulfuric acid, carbonic acid, and nitric acid. When it rains or snows, these acids are brought to Earth in what is called acid rain.

"During the course of the 20th century, the acidity of the air and acid rain has come to be recognized as a leading threat to the stability and quality of the Earth's environment. Most of this acidity is produced in the industrialized nations of the Northern Hemisphere—the United States, Canada, Japan, and most of the countries of Eastern and Western Europe.

"The effects of acid rain can be devastating to many forms of life, including human life. Its effects can be most vividly seen, however, in lakes, rivers, and streams and on vegetation. Acidity in water kills virtually all life forms. By the early 1990s, tens of thousands of lakes had been destroyed by acid rain. The problem has been most severe in Norway, Sweden, and Canada.

"The threat posed by acid rain is not limited by geographic boundaries, for prevailing winds carry the pollutants around the globe. For example, much research supports the conclusion that pollution from coal-powered electric generating stations in the Midwestern United States is the ultimate cause of the severe acid-rain problem in eastern Canada and the northeastern United States. Nor are the destructive effects of acid rain limited to the natural environment. Structures made of stone, metal, and cement have also been damaged or destroyed. Some of the world's great monuments, including the cathedrals of Europe and the Colosseum in Rome, have shown signs of deterioration caused by acid rain.

"Scientists use what is called the pH factor to measure the acidity or alkalinity of liquid solutions. On a scale from 0 to 14, the number 0 represents the highest level of acid and 14 the most basic or alkaline. A solution of distilled water containing neither acids nor alkalies, or bases, is designated 7, or neutral. If the pH level of rain falls below 5.5, the rain is considered acidic. Rainfalls in the eastern United States and in Western Europe often range from 4.5 to 4.0.

"Although the cost of such antipollution equipment as burners, filters, and chemical and washing devices is great, the cost in damage to the environment and human life is estimated to be much greater because the damage may be irreversible. Although preventative measures are being taken, up to 500,000 lakes in North America and more than 4 billion cubic feet (118 million cubic meters) of timber in Europe may be destroyed before the end of the 20th century." [2]

"Forestry is another cause for acidification. In the natural cycle, bases once taken up from the soil by trees eventually return once the trees decompose. The removal of large trees from the forest also removes large amounts of the bases that are needed for the acid-base balance of the forest. This slowly leads to acidification." [3]

Human health is not spared either. We eat food, drink water, and breathe air that has been exposed to acid deposition. This acidic air pollution can cause respiratory problems among children and asthmatics. Acid deposition can make its way into untreated drinking water supplies that cause food poisoning.

Although the focus of this book has been to change to an alkali-forming diet with pure alkaline water to resolve IC, let us not forget the air we breathe is acidic as well. The air we breathe contains sulfuric acid, nitric acid, and hydrochloric acid that need to be neutralized. In solving the IC puzzle, we cannot afford to ignore the big picture, for we are all a part of the world. In solving the IC puzzle, doctors, and researchers have been busy looking through a microscope when what we might need to do is view this problem with a "macroscope." The macroscope can be considered the symbol of a new way of seeing, understanding, and acting. We need to view our health holistically.

"Many urologists have come to the conclusion that we are dealing with a multifactorial disease entity that needs to be reclassified." [4]

"While much of the effort to treat interstitial cystitis has focused on identifying specific causes and markers for the disease, pain researchers at Johns Hopkins University in Baltimore have concluded that multi-faceted strategies are apparently needed to effectively treat the variety of underlying pain mechanisms that may exist in the same patient... A spectrum of different insults likely leads to chronic visceral pain in IC." [5]

Acid Air, Acid Rain
What I discovered to my amazement was that Norway and Sweden spend an equivalence of $40 to $50 million US dollars each year "liming" their lakes. What does liming their lakes entail? They are doing exactly what I have been discussing in this book. They add alkaline elements to an acidic environment to attain a neutralizing effect. They administer 300,000 tons of fine-grained limestone yearly into lakes, streams, and wetlands to raise the pH in surface water. Limestone, also known as calcium carbonate, an alkalizing element, is used to raise the water's pH level from a low 4 or 5 to a higher and life-sustaining pH of 6 to 8.

Just as taking an alkaline supplement instead of a

balanced alkali-forming diet/lifestyle is not recommended for IC, the liming solution is a shortsighted intervention rather than a long-term "cure." People and environments are too complex to be governed by one or two molecules.

Viewing IC Holistically

Traditionally, most Americans have been led to believe that one remedy could solve their health problems, that a visit to a doctor's office could cure what ails them, or that one type of treatment or a pill could improve their condition. In my healing process, I went to numerous medical doctors as well as holistic health care providers where I received pieces of this puzzle over many years for my recovery from IC.

When evaluating any disease it is vital that one examines the "big picture" and assesses all aspects of the person's life and environment. I doubt if very many IC sufferers have had a complete history and examination of their lives including their intake of foods, water and air quality, physical activity, vitamin, mineral and essential fatty acid sufficiency, stress levels and coping, allergies and system reviews.

What I have discovered with IC is there are many pieces to this puzzle—, that ones health needs to be viewed macroscopically. In solving the IC puzzle, I needed to consider the following: diet, including supplements and medications, water quality, air quality, allergies, stress, and lifestyle choices. These considerations needed to be evaluated from the perspective of pH and their correlation with each other. In addition, the systems that needed to be addressed for myself were the bladder, the gastrointestinal system, the liver, and the adrenal glands. These systems, too, needed to be evaluated with respect to pH and my body's balance.

All systems of the body affect ones pH. If a child has asthma, he would tend to be more acidic, since more carbon dioxide would be retained. If the kidneys were weak, one would see signs of acidosis as well. Each person with IC needs to evaluate the systems in their body, their external environment, diet, and lifestyle in order to resolve IC. Some people have a history of these acid-forming activities such as consuming alcohol, coffee, or smoking. Some people do none of these, but might live under considerable stress without having adequate coping skills. Some individuals have food allergies; others do not. My point is you will need to do your own self-inventory to determine what is causing your body's acid state.

I am of the belief that most persons with IC, if not all, have been treated with multiple courses of antibiotics. This history creates the LGS, allergies, and malnutrition that in turn tax the liver. These problems are acid-forming and need to be addressed. In addition, it has been documented that the majority of Americans eat an acid-forming diet, are deficient in their nutrition, and lead stressful lives. Converting to a nutritious alkali-forming diet with pure alkaline water and adequate supplementation plus finding ways to reduce stress and to heal the adrenal glands would be mandatory for persons with IC.

With respect to inhaling acidic air, I did not cover oxygen therapy. Remember that oxygen is an alkalizing element. There are oxygen therapies and ozone therapies that purify the air we breathe at home and in the office and provide the body with supplemental oxygen. Actually, ozone is simply pure, activated oxygen. I encourage the reader who wants not only relief from IC, but would like to live a *vigorous* life, to explore holistic applications of oxygen therapy. In addition, alkaline water does contain more available oxygen than ordinary water so drinking plenty of Microwater would boost the amount of ones daily oxygen intake.

I would also like to emphasize that consuming an acid-forming diet, drinking acid-forming beverages, and choosing an acid-forming lifestyle cannot merely be "treated" with an antacid or a supplement or two. I have witnessed after twenty years of nursing practice that this is a common history of persons who develop cancer. The body needs a healthy alkali-forming diet that provides the essential alkalizing elements, vitamins, minerals, fats, and trace elements.

Whether you understand all the systems in your body that are contributing to your body's level of acidity is not as important as understanding that maintaining an alkali-forming diet/lifestyle can help to neutralize the effects of living in an acidic environment.

Over the years that I suffered from IC, when I was not diagnosed accurately and wondered what was wrong with me, I got so discouraged and would ask myself why was I suffering and why me? I cursed, cried, and coped the best I could. Now that I am recovered, I can see that for me IC was truly a blessing. Having IC has been a humbling experience and has helped me to remember that in life there is suffering. It has made me more conscious of others who are hurting in this world. It motivated me to search for answers to my healing. In doing so, it has helped me learn so much.

In nursing school, we studied nutrition, and it has always been an interest of mine. Although I thought my diet was healthy, I learned I was making some wrong choices and had many deficiencies and so did my family.

Even though I do not have a crystal ball to see into the future, I am sure learning about the pH factor and its effect on my health will help prevent diseases, maybe even cancer. I know for most Americans pursuing an alkaline program put forth in this book may not be easy. However, for myself, because I endured so much pain from IC, I was highly motivated to make this change. For this I am grateful. I consider myself a spiritual person, but I found IC had renewed my sense of awe when I was reminded how the mystery of life is so beautifully interwoven. We really are one.

My wish in offering you this book about my discovery and recovery from IC is that it offers you a safe alternative approach for dealing with IC. Choosing an alkali-forming diet/lifestyle, healing the LGS, allergies, liver, and the adrenal glands has eliminated my suffering. I wish those of you who have endured so much pain for so long from IC have been given new hope. I welcome further exploration and study from persons with IC as well as caregivers and researchers who work with us regarding the effect of the pH factor and IC.

May you find renewed hope and inspiration in resolving IC.

Respectfully,

Amrit

Please visit my website at *http://www.holisticnurse.com* for resources and current developments in the treatment of interstitial cystitis.

[1] Adapted from http://www.science.mcmaster.ca/Biology/4S03/ar4.html

[2] Compton's Encyclopedia Online v3.0 © 1998 The Learning Company, Inc., http://www.comptons.com/encyclopedia/ARTICLES/0000/00013824_A.html

[3] http://www.vtek.chalmers.se/~v94zinn/liming.html

[4] Dr. Raymond A. Hurm, MD, *Urology Times*, Letter to the Editor, July 1999

[5] Dan Emerson, *Urology Times*, Jan, 2001

APPENDIX A — FOODS

In Appendix A, I have compiled a table of foods and categorized them according to their level of acidity or alkalinity. This appendix adapted from Dr. Baroody's *Alkalize or Die*. Attempt to eat a diet that contains 80 percent of your food choice from the alkali-forming categories.

Fruits

Highly Alkaline		
Cantaloupe	Dates (dried)	Figs (dried)
Lemons	Limes	Mangos
Melons (all varieties)	Papaya	Watermelon
Moderately Alkaline		
Apricots	Avocados	Bananas
Berries (except blueberries and cranberries)		Breadfruit
Cactus	Citron	Currants
Dates (fresh)	Figs (fresh)	Grapefruit
Grapes	Guavas	Kiwis
Kumquats	Nectarines	Passion Fruit
Peaches	Pears	Persimmons
Pineapple	Quince	Raisins
Tamarind	Tangerine	Umeboshi Plums
Slightly Alkaline		
Apples	Carob	Cherries
Olives (ripened and sun dried)		Oranges
Pomegranate	Raspberries	Strawberries
Neutral		
None Noted		
Slightly Acidic		
None Noted		
Moderately Acidic		
Blueberries	Cranberries	Plums
Prunes		
Highly Acidic		
None Noted		

(Overcooked fruit becomes acid-forming.)

Vegetables

Highly Alkaline		
Kelp	Parsley	Seaweed
Watercress		
Moderately Alkaline		
Asparagus	Carrots	Celery
Dandelion Greens	Endive	Escarole
Lettuce (all types)	Oyster Plant (Salsify)	Pumpkin
Rutabaga	Spinach	Squash
Slightly Alkaline		
Artichokes	Bamboo Shoots	Beets
Broccoli	Brussels Sprouts	Cabbage
Cauliflower	Chicory	Collards
Corn, sweet	Cucumbers	Daikon
Eggplant	Ginger (fresh)	Kale
Kohlrabi	Leeks	Lettuce, Iceberg
Mushrooms	Mustard greens	Okra
Onions	Parsnips	Peppers, Bell
Pickles	Potatoes	Swiss Chard
Taro (baked)	Tomatoes	Turnips
Radishes	Water Chestnuts	
Neutral		
Horseraddish	Rhubarb	Sauerkraut
Slightly Acidic		
None Noted		
Moderately Acidic		
None Noted		
Highly Acidic		
None Noted		

(Overcooked vegetables become acid-forming.)

188   Solving the Interstitial Cystitis Puzzle

Grains

Highly Alkaline		
None Noted		
Moderately Alkaline		
None Noted		
Slightly Alkaline		
None Noted		
Neutral		
Amaranth	Millet	Quinoa
Slightly Acidic		
Barley	Corn Meal	Rye
Spelt		
Moderately Acidic		
Basmati Rice	Brown Rice	Buckwheat
Oats	Whole Wheat	
Highly Acidic		
Wheat (bleached)	White Rice	

(All grains become neutral to slightly alkali-forming when sprouted.)

Beans

Highly Alkaline		
None Noted		
Moderately Alkaline		
None Noted		
Slightly Alkaline		
French Bean (fresh)	Green (fresh)	Lima (fresh)
Peas (fresh)	Snap (fresh)	String (fresh)
Neutral		
Soy Beans	Soy Cheese	Soy Milk
Tempeh	Tofu	
Slightly Acidic		
Aduki	Black	Broadbean
Garbanzo	Kidney	Lentils
Mung	Navy	Pinto
Red	White	
Moderately Acidic		
None Noted		
Highly Acidic		
None Noted		

(Acid-forming beans become slightly to moderately alkali-forming when sprouted.)

Other Starches

Highly Alkaline		
None Noted		
Moderately Alkaline		
Arrowroot Flour		
Slightly Alkaline		
Potatoes (all types)		
Neutral		
Essene Bread	Granola	
Slightly Acidic		
Bran	Popcorn (plain)	Popcorn with Butter
Unrefined Cold Cereals		Unrefined Crackers
Whole Grain Pastas		
Moderately Acidic		
Buckwheat Cereal (hot)		Corn Bread
Cream of Wheat (hot)	Popcorn with Butter and Salt	
Oat Bread	Oatmeal Cereal	Rice Bread
Rye Bread	Spelt Bread	Tapioca
Whole Grain Pastries	Popcorn with Salt	
Highly Acidic		
Refined Flours	Refined Pastas	Refined Pastries
Wheat Bread		

Nuts

Highly Alkaline		
None Noted		
Moderately Alkaline		
None Noted		
Slightly Alkaline		
Almonds	Coconut (fresh)	
Neutral		
Chestnuts	Pignolias	
Slightly Acidic		
Brazil	Cashews	Coconut (dried)
Filberts	Macadamia	Pecans
Pistachios	Walnuts	
Moderately Acidic		
Peanuts		
Highly Acidic		
None Noted		

Seeds

Highly Alkaline		
None Noted		
Moderately Alkaline		
Alfalfa (sprouted)	Chia (sprouted)	
Slightly Alkaline		
Radish (sprouted)		
Neutral		
Sesame (unsprouted)		
Slightly Acidic		
Pumpkin	Sunflower	
Moderately Acidic		
Wheat Germ		
Highly Acidic		
None Noted		

Meta

Highly Alkaline		
None Noted		
Moderately Alkaline		
None Noted		
Slightly Alkaline		
None Noted		
Neutral		
None Noted		
Slightly Acidic		
None Noted		
Moderately Acidic		
Crab	Fish (fins and scales)	Lobster
Oysters	Scallops	Shrimp
Highly Acidic		
Beef (organically grown)		
Chicken (organically grown)		Fish (other types)
Lamb	Pheasant	Pork
Rabbit	Turkey (organically grown)	
Turkey (wild)	Venison	

Animal Products

Highly Alkaline		
None Noted		

Moderately Alkaline		
None Noted		

Slightly Alkaline		
None Noted		

Neutral		
Butter (fresh unsalted)	Cow's milk (fresh, raw)	Cream (fresh, raw)
Egg Yolk	Goat's milk (raw)	
Lactobacillus Acidophilus		Lactobacillus Bifidus
Whey (cow's milk)	Whey (goat's milk)	Yogurt plain

Slightly Acidic		
Butter (fresh salted)	Butter (processed)	Cheese (crumbly)
Cheese (mild/medium)	Cottage Cheese	Cream (processed)
Egg Whites	Milk (cow's, homogenized)	
Milk (goat's homogenized)		

Moderately Acidic		
Cheese (sharp)	Custard	Sweetened Yogurt
Whole eggs		

Highly Acidic		
None Noted		

Oils

Highly Alkaline		
None Noted		
Moderately Alkaline		
None Noted		
Slightly Alkaline		
None Noted		
Neutral		
Almond	Avocado	Canola
Castor	Coconut	Corn
Margarine	Olive	Safflower
Sesame	Soy	Sunflower
Slightly Acidic		
None Noted		
Moderately Acidic		
None Noted		
Highly Acidic		
None Noted		

Sugars

Highly Alkaline		
None Noted		
Moderately Alkaline		
None Noted		
Slightly Alkaline		
Brown Rice Syrup	Dr. Bronner's Barley Malt Sweetener	
Honey (unprocessed)	Maguey	
Neutral		
Dried Sugar Cane Juice		
Slightly Acidic		
Barley malt syrup	Fructose	Honey (processed)
Maple syrup (unprocessed)		
Molasses (organic, unsulfured)		Milk sugar
Turbinado		
Moderately Acidic		
Maple syrup (processed)		
Molasses (processed, sulfured)		
Highly Acidic		
Beet sugar (processed, bleached)		
Cane sugar (white processed)		

Beverages

Highly Alkaline		
Alkaline Water	Fruit Juices (fresh)	Vegetable Juices
Moderately Alkaline		
Herbal Teas		
Slightly Alkaline		
None Noted		
Neutral		
None Noted		
Slightly Acidic		
Coffee Substitutes	Fruit Juice (naturally sweetened)	
Moderately Acidic		
Wine	Fruit Juice (sweetened with white sugar)	
Highly Acidic		
Beer	Caffeine Drinks	Carbonated Drinks
Coffee	Liquor	Soft Drinks
Tea (black)		

Condiments

Highly Alkaline		
Agar-Agar	Cayenne Pepper	

Moderately Alkaline		
Bay leaves	Chives	
Dr. Bronner's Mineral Bouillon		Garlic
Gelatin (plain, unsugared with fruit or vegetables)		
Marjoram	Vegetable Salt	

Slightly Alkaline		
Apple Cider Vinegar (raw, unprocessed)		Basil
Caraway Seed	Celery Seed	Cloves
Coriander	Cumin Seed	Curry Powder
Dill Leaves	Fennel Seed	Ginger (powdered)
Ketchup (natural)	Miso	Oregano
Paprika	Potassium (Bio-salt)	Rosemary
Sage	Sea Salt	
Sweet Brown Rice Vinegar		Tamari
Tarragon	Thyme	Vanilla Extract

Neutral		
Anise	Brewer's Yeast	Cinnamon
Distilled Water	Nutritional Yeast	Soy Sauce

Slightly Acidic		
Gelatin (mixed with water)		Mustard (dried spice)
Mustard (stone ground, natural)		Nutmeg

Moderately Acidic		
Gelatin (mixed with sugar)		Ketchup (refined)
Mayonnaise (refined with sugar)		Soy sauce (processed)

Highly Acidic		
Mustard (refined)	Salt (refined, white)	White Vinegar

APPENDIX B — LIFESTYLE CHOICES

Alkali-Forming Lifestyle

Alkali-forming diet	Laughter
Counseling or therapy can reduce stress	Adequate alkaline water intake 6-8 glasses per day
Yoga improves breathing	Deep breathing
Silence	Chew food thoroughly
Parasite and yeast elimination program (Clear® supplement)	Essential fiber in diet decreases constipation
Adequate nutrition with essential vitamins, minerals and fatty acids	Hobbies that relax the body and mind
Meditation	Mineral baths
Allergy testing and elimination to decrease inflammation	Massage helps clean the lymphatic system
Aromatherapy (lavender essential oil can be added to a bath, handkerchief or a few drops diluted in almond oil for a relaxing massage)	Green foods high in chlorophyll removes toxins from the body and increase magnesium and oxygenation (spirulina, chlorella, alfalfa, barley grass; look for Green Magma™ and/or Kyo-green™ on the market)
Saunas help eliminate toxins, but be sure to replace lost minerals and fluids with juices and alkaline water	Enteric-coated probiotics (lactobacillus bifidus and lactobacillus acidophilus)
Liver/ gallbladder flush (bile: pH 8 from the liver helps to digest food which enhances ones nutritional state and the liver helps to detoxify the body of harmful chemicals)	Detoxification programs (consult a holistic health care provider)

Alkali-Forming Lifestyle

Oxygen therapies	Eat moderately
Reflexology helps to strengthen and rebalance body systems	Biofeedback (learn to modify responses to stress)
Sodium bicarbonate	Potassium bicarbonate
Kidney flushes (consult a holistic health care provider)	Attend to your spiritual needs as well as physical and mental
Relaxing walks in nature	A day at a health spa
Pets have been shown to reduce stress and blood pressures in their owners	Homeopathics and appropriate supplements that support acid-alkali balance
Adequate rest and relaxation every day	Acupuncture to assist in balancing the acid-alkali balance
Colonics and enemas are good for detoxification (consult a holistic health care provider)	Mild to moderate fasting (fruit or vegetable juice fasting) can help rebalance acid-alkali balance
Relaxing environment such as the use of natural-scented candles, incense and flowers (provided they are not allergens) water fountains, wind chimes, pleasant colors, inspiring artwork and music, aquariums etc.	Mild to moderate exercise every day (walking, swimming, or bike riding are a good start, but see a health care provider if you have medical conditions or are over 40 years old before starting such a program)
Sunlight (exposure for 30 minutes to two hours a day benefits the adrenal glands; these glands help us regulate our stress fight or flight response)	Ozone air purifiers (placed in a room they will eliminate fungi, bacteria, molds pollutants and chemicals in the air)

Acid-Forming Lifestyle

Cosmetics, shampoo, soap, hair dye, makeup not organically based since these are absorbed through the skin and scalp	98% of prescription and over the counter drugs produce acid forming reactions
Stress (situations that cause anxiety, anger, fear, disappointment; even success can still be stressors)	Decreased pancreatic fluids (pancreatic fluids are alkaline with a pH of 8.4 to 8.9 and help to neutralize acids)
Respiratory conditions (carbon dioxide an acid is retained and not enough oxygen is absorbed)	Gallbladder and liver diseases from over-consumption, obesity, alcohol and drugs
Drinking acidic water	Kidney disease
Increased hydrochloric acid in the stomach; increases acid load in the body	Alcohol causes excretion of nutrients in the urine especially calcium and magnesium
Sedentary lifestyle	Over-exercising
Parasites and Infections	Allergies and inflammatory conditions
Toxins/chemicals in food and environment	Salt (too much sodium causes potassium to be excreted)
Sugar	Overcooked foods
Tired adrenal glands from too much stress, caffeine and sugar	Caffeine causes the kidneys to excrete alkaline elements
Thyroid disease	Leaky Gut Syndrome
Refined and processed foods	Tobacco (smoking or chewing)
Antibiotics destroy normal gut flora	Air pollution decreases oxygen, an alkaline element

Acid-Forming Lifestyle

Constipation (toxic acid wastes are reabsorbed into the system instead of eliminated)	Malnutrition and anemia (lack of essential vitamins, minerals and essential fatty acids)
Sluggish lymphatic system related to sedentary life style and decreased water intake	Shallow breathing and holding the breath causes the retention of carbon dioxide, an acid

APPENDIX C — MINERALS

Solving the Interstitial Cystitis Puzzle

The following are some tables, which at a glance list the following sources of foods high in certain alkalizing elements:

Calcium

(1000mg RDA for a 150 lb adult)

2 oz	Cheese	350mg
1-cup	Yogurt	300mg
3 oz	Salmon	200mg
4	Sardines	200mg
1-cup	Soybeans (cooked)	175mg
1-cup	Collards (cooked)	150mg
1-T	Molasses	140mg
1 oz	Almonds	80mg

Iron

(10 mg RDA for a 150 lb adult)

3 oz.	Oysters	12mg
1-cup	Fortified Whole Cereal	10mg
1-cup	Soybeans (cooked)	9mg
4 oz.	Liver	8mg
1-cup	Lentils (cooked)	7mg
½ -cup	Spinach (cooked)	3mg
1T	Molasses	3mg
8 oz.	Prune Juice	3mg
10	Prunes	2mg

Potassium

(2500mg for a 150 lb adult)

1	Papaya	800mg
1-cup	Prune Juice	700mg
6 oz.	Carrot Juice	700mg
½	Avocado	600mg
5	Peach Halves (dried)	600mg
1 T	Molasses	585mg
10	Dates	550mg
5	Pear Halves (dried)	500mg
1-cup	Cantaloupe	500mg
1-cup	Orange Juice	500mg
10 halves	Apricots (dried)	500mg
1	Banana	450mg
1-cup	2% Chocolate Milk	400mg
1-cup	Tomato Juice	400mg
1-cup	Pineapple Juice	350mg
1-cup	Grape Juice	350mg
1-cup	Grapefruit Juice	350mg
1	Mango	300mg
1	Tomato	250mg
1-cup	Tomato Soup	250mg

Magnesium

(350 mg RDA for 150 lb adult)

1 oz.	Pumpkin Seeds	150mg
1-cup	Soybeans (cooked)	150mg
1 square	Rye Crisp	140mg
½ -cup	100% Bran Cereal	140mg
1-cup	Black Beans (cooked)	120mg
¼-cup	Toasted Wheat Germ	100mg
1-cup	Millet (cooked)	100mg
3 oz.	Oysters (steamed)	100mg
3 oz.	Halibut (baked)	100mg
1 oz.	Almonds (dry roasted)	100mg
1 oz.	Sunflower Seeds	100mg
1-cup	Navy Beans (cooked)	100mg
1-cup	Lima Beans (cooked)	100mg
1	Prickly Pear	90mg
1 T	Molasses	50mg

Sodium

(2000mg RDA for 150 lb adult)

Sodium is found in virtually all foods and table salt (examples are one burrito or one cup of chili contains 1000mg of sodium.) As stated earlier the average American diet is rarely deficient in this element therefore we will not review the food sources. It should be mentioned again, however, that an excess of sodium might lead to the loss of potassium in the urine.

APPENDIX D — MEAL SUGGESTIONS

Breakfast

ʖ Granola Cereal (cereal made from oatmeal, seeds, nuts, and dried fruit): Try calcium fortified vanilla soy or rice milk on the cereal for a change

ʖ French toast made with sprouted grain bread or rice or soy flour bread, egg, vanilla soy or rice milk, and maple syrup with pat of butter

ʖ Fruit "Sundae" made with banana, grapes, strawberries topped with yogurt, wheat germ, and chopped pecans

ʖ Fruit smoothie (blender drink with favorite fruits, juice, ice, and yogurt)

ʖ Dish of mixed dried fruit like papaya, mango, figs, prunes, and dates with almonds, pumpkin and sunflower seeds

ʖ Vegetable omelet with fresh fruit

ʖ Sprouted grain bread toasted with almond butter and organic fruit jelly, jam, or honey

ʖ Vanilla yogurt, fruit, and almonds

ʖ One scrambled egg with free-range turkey sausage and fresh fruit

ʖ Fruit juices: orange juice, pineapple juice, papaya juice, prune juice, tomato juice, grapefruit juice, apricot nectar, and peach or pear nectar [1]

Lunch

- Vegetable Salad with rye crackers and cheese

- Tossed salad, baked potato, and butter

- Vegetable soup with rye crackers and cheese

- Pita bread sandwich with free-range chicken or turkey, vegetables, sprouts, and dressing

- Whole grain sprouted bread with almond or nut butter and sprouts or lettuce

- Fruit salad with yogurt, cheese, or cottage cheese

- Vegetable or free-range chicken tacos or tostada with tomatoes, lettuce, onion, guacamole, and soy cheddar cheese

- Minestrone soup with cheese

- Tomato or corn soup with coleslaw

- Split pea soup with salad

- Vegetable quiche and fruit dessert

- Greek salad

- Vegetarian chili with corn bread

- Gazpacho with rye bread and butter

- Veggie and almond butter sandwich on sprouted grain bread with vegetable juice

Dinner

Serve a relish tray with mixed raw vegetable strips at every evening meal.

- Broiled salmon with steamed carrots-broccoli and pumpkin pie

- Veggie burger with a baked potato and tossed salad

- Fettuccini with broccoli floret and tossed salad

- Free-range turkey with sweet potatoes and zucchini

- Vegetable salad, herbed mashed potatoes, steamed broccoli

- Tofu with vegetables

- Tuna burger with baked potato and tossed salad

- Salmon pasta salad

- Vegetable chow mien

- Stir-fry vegetables with brown rice

- Broiled garlic shrimp with cabbage salad and steamed green beans with slivered almonds

- Spaghetti using spinach rice pasta with tomato sauce and Parmesan cheese with tossed salad (Try the Italian soy "meatless" mix in the sauce; it is very good.)

Snacks

All nuts and chips should be salt-free or low salt.

- Vegetable sticks with ranch dressing, hummus, or nut butters

- Salt-free corn chips with guacamole

- Rice cakes with nut butter

- Vegetable juice

- Nut butter cookie

- Fresh fruit

- Handful of salt-free almonds and seeds with mixed dried fruits

- Rye crisp with soy cheese

- Green drinks (Magma™)

- Oatmeal, fig, or raisin cookie

- Popcorn

Troublesome Foods

Tannic acid is found in the following foods and are usually not well tolerated by persons with IC with an acid-alkali imbalance: chocolate, grapes, red and white wines, cola drinks, black and pekoe teas, and coffee.

Citric and malic acid are found in tomatoes; they might worsen symptoms in IC.

Vinegar and items that contain vinegar may cause a worsening of IC symptoms due to the acetic acid found in vinegar.

For those individuals who like to take Vitamin C (ascorbic acid) supplements and can not tolerate it; consider taking buffered vitamin C. A company called Allergy Research Group makes a good buffered vitamin C with the following contents: one heaping teaspoon contains Vitamin C 2,350mg buffered with calcium 450 mg, Magnesium 250 mg, and Potassium 99mg.

1. Persons with IC report a worsening of symptoms after eating "acidic foods" such as citrus fruits. Citrus fruits are actually alkali-forming, however they do contain citric acid, which may be troublesome. I found by starting my alkali-forming diet with mostly vegetables and adding citric fruits slowly when I was more alkaline, I was able to tolerate citric fruits once my urine pH was 7.

APPENDIX E — RESOURCES & SUPPLIERS

Sodium bicarbonate is baking soda and can be purchased at a grocery store.

Sodium citrate, USP. This can be ordered from health food stores. Make sure you order USP, US Pharmacopoeia grade.

Probiotics: Buy enteric-coated (EC) capsules that are found in the refrigerated section of your health food store.

Potassium bicarbonate, USP, is only available from a chemical supply house. I purchased mine from Chem-Lab Supplies on the Internet. Make sure you order USP, US Pharmacopoeia grade.

Chem-Lab Supplies

13814 Inglewood Ave

Hawthorne, CA 90250

(310) 973-2391

Web Address: http://www.chemlab.com

Herbal Formula Clear®

to order call

(800) 69AWARE or (800) 692-9273

Mention Distributor Number 11157401

Web Address: http://www.holisticnurse.com/topics/aware/

Corporate Headquarters

Awareness Corporation

3300 N Central Ave

Suite 2350

Phoenix, AZ 85012

(602) 265-1900

(800) 810-9964 (US and Canada)

(530) 292-3370 (international)

Web Address: http://www.awarecorp.com.

AlkaLife®

A 1.2 oz. bottle lasts about two months and costs about $18.95.

Sang Whang Enterprises, Inc.

8445 SW 148 Dr

Miami, FL 33158

 (888) 261-0870

Web Address: http://www.alkalife.com

E-Mail Address: sang@alkalife.com

BHI Homeopathic Remedies

Manufactured and distributed by:

Heel Incorporated

11600 Cochiti Road SE

Albuquerque, NM 87123-3376

(800) 621-7644

(505) 293-3843

Web Address: http://www.heelbhi.com

E-Mail Address: info@heelbhi.com

Slippery Stuff® Gel

Distributed by

Wallace-O'Farrell

11302 164th Street East

Puyallup, WA 98374

In North America the telephone numbers are

(800) 759-7883 or (206) 845-6633

A web site that sells Slippery Stuff Gel is

http://www.take-care.com/preg/physicianrecommended.html

Nambudripad Allergy Research Foundation

6714 Beach Blvd

Buena Park, CA 90621

(714) 523-0800

http://www.naet.com/

Water Ionizer

The Bluestone Group

(412) 833-9640

http://www.bluestonegroup.com/

American Holistic Nurses Association

PO Box 2130

Flagstaff, AZ 86003-2130

(800) 278-2462

http://www.ahna.org

American Holistic Medical Association

6728 Old McLean Village Drive

McLean, VA 22101

Tel: (703) 556-9245

Fax: (703) 556-8729

holistmed@aol.com

Interstitial Cystitis Association

http://www.ichelp.org

Interstial Cystitis Network

http://www.ic-network.com

APPENDIX F — SUPPLEMENTS

Sodium bicarbonate: for IC symptoms, oral dose ¼ teaspoon to ½ teaspoon mixed in 4 oz of water every hour or two until IC symptoms abate

Potassium bicarbonate, USP, should not be taken by itself. Recommended to mix with sodium bicarbonate 4:1 or 8:1 (four parts sodium bicarbonate to one part potassium bicarbonate or eight parts sodium bicarbonate to one part potassium bicarbonate)

Sodium and potassium bicarbonate mixture (4:1 or 8:1 depending on your tolerance for potassium): for inflammatory conditions, oral dose ¼ to ½ teaspoon mixed in 4 oz of water three to four times a day preferably ½ hour before a meal or two hours after a meal

Sodium citrate, USP: for sustained relief from IC, oral dose ½ to ¾ teaspoon mixed in 4 oz of water twice a day

EC Probiotics: Oral dose daily, as recommended by product label

Herbal Formula Clear® anti-parasitic and anti-fungal: one each morning on an empty stomach with water only

AlkaLife® is a patented alkaline concentrate. Mix 2 drops of AlkaLife solution in an 8-oz glass of water changes ordinary drinking water to high pH alkaline drinking water.

Chelated Vitamin / Mineral supplements, preferably liquid and total Essential Fatty Acid (EFA), liquid or capsule (flaxseed oil, evening primrose oil, borage seed oil, and lecithin)

BHI Homeopathic Remedies for allergy flare-ups: allergy homeopathic and inflammation homeopathic. These two homeopathics worked fantastic in eliminating IC flare-ups when I was allergic to foods I consumed.

MSM (methylsulfonylmethane): for inflammation and anti-parasitic, the suggested dosage is 250mg to 750mg of MSM taken three times per day in divided doses with meals.

Bromelain: For inflammation, suggested dosage is 500mg taken two to four times per day apart from meals for inflammation. It should not be taken by pregnant women or persons with bleeding disorders.

Papain: For inflammation, suggested dosage is 200mg to 300mg with or immediately following meals, upon rising, and before bedtime. It should not be taken by pregnant women or persons with bleeding disorders.

Pantothenic Acid: suggested dosages: for stress, take 100mg per day; for allergies, take 500mg three times a day; for Chronic Fatigue Syndrome, take 500mg twice a day

Milk Thistle: as a liver remedy, suggested dosage is one capsule up to three times daily.

APPENDIX G — SUMMARY OF MY REGIMEN

Weeks One and Two

§ I started on an alkali-forming diet with distilled water and began testing my urine pH while keeping an IC food diary.

§ I eliminated all bladder irritants such as coffee, wine, all over the counter drugs, supplements, and herbs.

§ A holistic health care provider tested me for food and environmental allergies.

§ I eliminated certain allergenic foods and continued a food log for the foods I could comfortably eat. If I got a flare-up, I used my BHI homeopathic remedies for allergy and inflammation, which eliminated any IC pains from the food allergy in about ten to fifteen minutes.

§ I noticed the better alkalized I was that my IC symptoms diminished.

§ By the end of week two, I was ninety percent pain-free.

Weeks Three and Four

- I started taking two EC probiotics (Jarrow Formulas™) every morning and started to drink alkaline water.

- I introduced the supplement sodium bicarbonate and potassium bicarbonate mixture in a four-to-one ratio. I only took one or two doses every other week during this time when I had flare-up that did not subside with homeopathics.

Weeks Five and Six

- I began to take chelated liquid vitamin and mineral supplements and a total essential fatty acid supplement every day.

- I started on a bowel program to repair the LGS and eliminate parasites by taking one Clear® capsule every morning. Parasites such as yeast and certain "bad" bacteria in the bowel are very acidifying and are common problems, especially after antibiotics.

Weeks Seven and Eight

- I did a gallbladder/liver flush.

- I started to take moderate walks twice a day to increase circulation and help eliminate acids.

- By the end of week eight, I was one hundred percent pain-free and was able to tolerate all citrus foods and spicy foods. My food allergies were ninety percent eliminated by this time.

INDEX

Symbols

A

B

F

258   Solving the Interstitial Cystitis Puzzle

O

IC Diary

Time	Void	pH	Food
6:00			
6:30			
7:00			
7:30			
8:00			
8:30			
9:00			
9:30			
10:00			
10:30			
11:00			
11:30			
12:00			
12:30			
1:00			
1:30			
2:00			
2:30			
3:00			
3:30			
4:00			
4:30			
5:00			
5:30			

Date:

Pain (0-10)	Miscellaneous

Notes

Solving the Interstitial Cystitis Puzzle

Notes

Notes

278   Solving the Interstitial Cystitis Puzzle

Notes

Notes

_____

_____

_____

_____

_____

_____

_____

_____

_____

_____

_____

_____

_____

_____

_____

_____

_____

_____

Notes

Notes

_____

_____

_____

_____

_____

_____

_____

_____

_____

_____

_____

_____

_____

_____

_____

_____

_____

_____

_____

Notes

Order Form

For additional copies of this book:

Solving the Interstitial Cystitis Puzzle
My Story of Discovery and Recovery

ISBN: 0-9710869-1-5

Send cheque or money order in the amount of $22.95 each to:

Holistic Life Enterprises

9461 Charleville Blvd Ste 198

Beverly Hills, CA 90212-3017

Name: _____

Address: _____

_____

City: _____

State: _____ Postal Code: _____ - _____

Make cheques payable to Holistic Life Enterprises

MasterCard   or   Visa   (Please circle appropriate type.)

_____ _____ _____ _____   exp. ____ / ____

Signature _____ Date _____

Order Form

For additional copies of this book:

Solving the Interstitial Cystitis Puzzle
My Story of Discovery and Recovery

ISBN: 0-9710869-1-5

Send cheque or money order in the amount of $22.95 each to:

Holistic Life Enterprises

9461 Charleville Blvd Ste 198

Beverly Hills, CA 90212-3017

Name: _____

Address: _____

_____

City: _____

State: _____ Postal Code: _____ - _____

Make cheques payable to Holistic Life Enterprises

MasterCard   or   Visa (Please circle appropriate type.)

_____ _____ _____ _____   exp. ____ / ____

Signature _____ Date _____